Fast for Focus

Your Fasting Guide to a Longer Life - Reclaim Your Health and Energy Beat Stress & Boost Your Mood

Alex Locklear

Table of content:

Introduction

Remember the time you walked into a room and had no idea why you were there? How about when you tried really hard to remember a name but just couldn't?

Every once in a while, we all have those little brain hiccups, but after age 40, they can feel like they happen more often. The feeling that our brains aren't as sharp as they used to be starts out as a small change. Some changes are normal as you get older, but they don't have to lead to forgetting and mental fog all the time. Indeed, being aware of these changes is the first thing that gives us the power to take care of our brain health.

Truth be told, as we age, our brains do change in some ways. It might take a moment or two longer for our memory to retrieve knowledge, and it might take a little longer to think about complicated ideas or do several things at once. But here's the thing: these changes don't need to scare you. Imagine that they are your brain's changes as it adapts to decades of information and events. The parts of our brain that deal with knowledge and language actually get bigger as we age. Shouldn't we be happy about that?

Of course, as we get older, we are more likely to get some diseases, like mild cognitive decline or Alzheimer's disease, which is so sad. Also, the way our bodies handle our moods can change, which can make us more likely to feel down sometimes. You should be aware of these risks, but there is good news: they are NOT certain to happen. The way we live has a huge effect on how our brain health changes over time. Imagine that you don't take care of your car and never change the oil. Then you shouldn't be shocked when the engine starts to sputter. Our brains need the   same   kind   of   care!

With this book, you'll learn how to fix your brain better than anyone else. We'll talk about the cool science behind how fasting, what you eat, and other healthy habits can make those gears inside your body shine. This chapter may talk about some of the truths about getting older brains, but remember that it's also the start of the story of brain resilience and strength.

Why People Over 40?

Brain Health Changes Around Midlife. Isn't this a strange and wonderful time? We have enough years under our belts to be wise, but the road ahead still feels like it's full of options. We're an interesting mix of old and new ideas and energy. But here's something that a lot of us don't talk about enough: the small changes that are happening in our brains and bodies. Learning about these changes isn't meant to make us feel down; it's meant to give us a whole new level of health freedom.

Let us talk about hormones, mainly for women. For women getting close to menopause, changes in estrogen levels and their final drop have a big effect on both their brains and their monthly cycles. Estrogen is good for brain health because it affects memory, happiness, and even the making of neurotransmitters.

So that mental roller coaster some of us go through? Not just in our heads; it has to do with our bodies as well. What's more, information is power. We can deal with these changes by making changes to our lifestyles and, for some women, by getting medical help.

Think of our bodies in midlife as ledgers, not just chemicals.

Years of what we've eaten, how much sleep we've had (or not gotten), and the stress we've been under start to add up. We may not have noticed the effects of those late nights with pizza in our 20s right away, but our brains kept very detailed records.

In the same way, having a job that makes us feel stressed out every day has an effect. This is where long-term illnesses like diabetes, high blood pressure, and bad cholesterol levels can start to show up and hurt our brain health even more.

Today is a good day to remind you that adulthood is NOT too late. What a great way to wake up, in fact. As adults, we know that fad diets and quick-fix plans to get fit don't lead to real happiness. We still want to make long-lasting changes to what we eat, how we move, and how we deal with the things that make life stressful. In this case, fasting and living a healthy life together have a huge effect. It's kind of like cleaning your brain and body for spring.

We are finally ready to spend money on preventative health care that will give us the energy and mental clarity to really do well in our middle years and beyond.

The Power of Fasting: It's Not Just for Losing Weight If the word "fasting" makes you think of juice cleanses or extreme diets that you can't stick to, you need to change the way you think about it. Fasting has been around for a very long time and has roots in many different spiritual and cultural beliefs. But new research shows that it's more than just a short-lived weight-loss trend. It's a powerful way to help our bodies and brains fix themselves naturally.

Imagine that your cells are small, busy towns. Over time, as we eat, they make trash and gather old, broken-down "machinery."

When you fast, it's like pressing the reset button. In a process called autophagy, which means "self-eating," it gives your cell cleanup crew a chance to catch up. This process gets rid of the junk so that new, healthy cell parts can be formed. Brain-Derived Neurotrophic Factor is the next one. It helps neurons grow, connect, and stay strong, like magic fertilizer for your brain.

Interestingly, fasting seems to make more BDNF.

Our brains are very demanding parts of our bodies. An unfair amount of our energy resources are used by them. The brain learns to work better when you fast. It learns how to switch power sources and better meet its energy needs. As a result? Not just a smaller waist (though that can be a nice bonus), but a mind that is clearer and smarter and better able to deal with problems.

New findings are still being made in the study of fasting and brain health, but the proof is very strong. There are signs that it might help with a lot of different conditions, from slowing down cognitive decline and preventing damage from strokes to improving happiness and thinking more clearly.

No matter what experts find out next, one thing is certain: fasting isn't just about the number on the scale. It's about giving your brain the tools it needs to do well now and, in the years, to come. You don't just want to fit into skinny pants; you want to live a full, healthy life for decades to come.

Chapter 1: Your Amazing, Aging Brain

How the brain changes as we age: What's normal and what's not

To be honest, your brain can feel like an old computer from time to time: it knows what it's doing but sometimes has problems. When we are in our mid-40s and older, we often walk into a place and ask ourselves, "Wait, why am I here?"

We all have our favorite phrases to use when we're "getting older," having a senior moment, or just "getting older." What's going on inside that great control center, though?

First, the good news: those short-lived memory problems and slower thinking speeds are a normal part of getting older. Think of it like the well-worn path through your yard. You know the way, but there may be fewer flowers in bloom, and it takes a little longer to get around. It's normal for things to change now that your brain has been used a lot.

Then, what's normal as your brain grows up?

• Less big and slower: As you age, your brain gets a little smaller, just like the rest of your body. The prefrontal cortex and the hippocampus, which handle learning, complex thinking, and memory, are two areas that are most likely to be affected. This means that you may not process knowledge as quickly as you did when you were in your 20s.

• Multitasking Mess: Remember how you used to be able to do a lot of things at once? It takes a little more work to switch between things as you get older. You might find that focusing on one thing at a time helps you get things done faster and better.

• Name Games: You'll have more "tip-of-the-tongue" moments where that known word is just out of reach. It has to do with the fact that your brain is getting information a little more slowly. The word is there; it just needs a little more time to come out.

Note: These changes are normal and won't stand out too much. You are still very smart, but your operating system is a little more "seasoned." But sometimes our brains need a little extra help.

Let's talk about some things that aren't normal for older people: Warning Signs: When "senior moments" Could Be More

• Disruptive Memory Loss: Can't remember where you left your car? A lot of the time losing things? That's pretty normal. But you should see a doctor if memory loss gets in the way of your daily life, like forgetting how to make a favorite meal or how to get to a place you've been before.

We all have bad days, but if you or someone you care about notices that your attitude changes often, your mood swings are too big, or you're becoming less interested in things, it's time for a checkup.

• Confusion Central: If normal jobs seem too hard or you get lost in places you've been before, it's better to rule out medical causes than to say you're "just getting older."

The part that gives you power: you can make your brain stronger! Okay, we accept that as we age, our brains change in some ways.

But here's the cool thing about your brain: it can change very easily! It will stay stronger as long as you use it and take good care of it, like a muscle. In the same way that it seems impossible to go to the gym and not feel better, your brain doesn't work the same way. Here is where the fun of fasting comes in.

According to new research, fasting doesn't just affect our waistlines; it can also help the brain fix itself and feel fresh again. It's like pressing the "reset" button on those memory pathways. It improves your attention and might even protect those precious brain cells from getting older. Yes, that's the kind of power we all want as we age.

Something to cheer you up

Being aware of "normal" changes makes getting older a lot less scary. You should not fight the way your brain is changing; instead, you should work with it. And the fact that doing good things, like fasting, can help your brainpower is just plain inspiring! You are about to learn how to use a powerful tool to protect and improve your most valuable asset: your amazing, aging brain.

Memory Loss, Loss of Focus, and Those Brain Fog Moments Are Common Problems

Let's see how many of us have been there: you're having a great chat when all of a sudden, the person's name leaves your mind. Or, you have a million things going on in your mind at once, and all of a sudden, that important thing you were supposed to do is gone. Your brain can feel like it's going through molasses some days, too. It can be slow, foggy, and not fully working. Sense a pattern?

One thing about getting older is that these blips and fuzzy times happen more often. It makes us think that maybe this is just "how it is" or even a reason to be worried. You're not alone, that's good news! Now let's break these problems down and talk about why they happen.

Challenge #1: Making Memories Go Wrong

Everyone has had that "tip-of-the-tongue" moment when they can't think of a word or name. There are a few reasons why these annoying memory slips happen more often as we age:

• Slower Retrieval: The brain processes you use all the time, like the ones that remember your name, are very fast. It takes longer for your brain to find new information or memories that you don't use as often. If you want to find something, it's like choosing between searching an organized file closet and rummaging through an attic. Either way, you'll find it faster.

• Wiring that is "noisy": Our brains are quite busy. A little more of this "noise" can be heard as we age. Remember when you were trying to tune in a weak radio station? That annoying static can make it harder to lock on to the signal.

Challenge #2: Focus Fade-Out

Do you remember when you could work on a job for hours on end? It may seem like your attention span is getting shorter these days. Why does this take place?

• The Multitasking Myth: We think we're great at doing many things at once, but our brains work best when they're focused on one thing at a time. If you jump from one job to another quickly, you'll quickly lose your focus energy as you get older.

• Tiredness of the Mind: An older brain can handle more stress. Your attention span is like a battery. It doesn't hold a charge all day like it used to after years of use.

Challenge #3: Welcome to Brain Fog City

Sometimes your thoughts are so fuzzy that you feel like you're putting a blanket over your head. That's brain fog. It is annoying! This could be what's causing the haze:

• Sleep Debt: Getting enough good sleep is important for organizing your thoughts and getting rid of "gunk" in your brain. Not getting enough sleep is like telling your brain's recycling plant to go on strike.

• worry Overload: Long-term worry floods the brain with cortisol, which makes it hard to concentrate and think straight.

• Hidden Causes: Brain fog can sometimes be a sign of not getting enough nutrients, changes in hormones, or even side effects from medications. If it doesn't go away, you should talk to your doctor about it.

The Part That Gives You Power: These Brain Blips Don't Own You!

You might feel down about these problems, but here's the thing: you don't have to go along with them. The first step to taming brain blips is to figure out "why" they happen. Also, guess what? One really cool thing about fasting is that it can help your brain in all of these ways.

Here's a sneak peek at what's to come:

• Memory Rescue: Fasting can help clear out the "cobwebs" in your mind and make it easier to remember things.

• Laser-Like Focus: Some research shows that fasting can block out unwanted noise, making it easier to focus and stay on task.

• Getting Rid of the Fog: Fasting is like cleaning out your mind, it helps get rid of the fog and makes it easier to think clearly. Shift your thoughts, shift your brain.

Stop seeing memory lapses or fuzzy moments as signs of getting worse and start seeing them for what they are: chances! They're signs that it's time to do something to improve your brain. Think of those spikes as your brain saying, "Hey, give me some of that fasting magic!" We'll talk more about HOW to do it in later chapters, but for now, stop being upset. At any age, this is about taking charge and using your brain to its fullest!

The Good News: Your brain can change a lot.

Think of your brain not as a fragile old thing, but as a strong machine that is always getting better. We've believed for too long that our brains reach their peak in our twenties and then slowly start to decline after that. I have bad news: that's not true! That myth about the aging brain is being busted wide open by science, which is very powerful.

Neuroplasticity is the word for this amazing trait. It means that your brain can change, adapt, and make new links throughout its life. Think of it this way: the parts of our brain that we use a lot get stronger, like climbing trails that have been used a lot. That being said, you can definitely break new ground and explore uncharted mental territory at any age if you put in the work.

How does the brain change?

In the best way possible, let's get serious! This is what happens in your brain when it can adapt:

• Growth Mindset, Meet Brain Growth: It turns out that the way we think can change the shape of our brains. New brain cells are made when you focus on learning and challenges. This is called neurogenesis. Welcome to the new paths!

As you learn something new, you make stronger links between brain cells (neurons) and make new ones. This is called "rewiring." This is the process of your brain rebuilding itself.

• Use It or (Kind of) Lose It: Brain pathways that are healthy are like muscles: the more you use them, the stronger they get. If you don't take care of them for too long, they will get weaker. This is why difficult brain tasks are so important as we age.

What Does THIS Mean for YOUR Brain as It Ages?

The crazy good news is that it's never too late to work out your brain! Taking on new tasks, like mastering a skill, learning a language, or even just walking around the block a few times in a different way, helps your brain adapt and make new connections.

But there's something extra special that happens when we fast and give our minds a task...

Fasting: A Speed Booster for Brain Improvement

Remember how we talked about autophagy (which cleans up cells) and BDNF (which helps brain cells grow) as brain healing powerhouses? Both get a boost from fasting! In short:

• Calling all spring cleaners! Fasting can help your brain get rid of old or broken cells and other cell junk. You can think of it as getting rid of mental clutter to make room for new, better brain paths.

• Fresh Brain Cells? Please say yes! Studies have shown that fasting can make the body make more BDNF. More BDNF means that more brain cells could grow, which would help you learn better and remember things better.

With real people and real results

Science is cool, but how does this show up in real life? People who fast often say they feel mentally sharper, with clearer thinking, better memory recall, and the annoying brain fog starting to lift. It's not just about stopping decline; it's about helping people of all ages reach their full potential.

The "Use It or Lose It" Test for Your Brain

Think about all the things you put off because you said, "I'm getting too old to learn that." Well, guess what? That's a prediction that comes true! Let's think of getting older as a chance to use your brain's power in even more exciting ways. For starters, here are some thoughts to get your mind going:

• Learn a new language. Learning a new language is like eating a superfood for your brain—it forces it to make new links.

• Get It Out: Did you play music when you were a kid? It works your brain in a special way whether you pick it up again or start from scratch.

• Get lost on purpose: Don't always use GPS when you drive. New routes are a great way to improve your spatial direction skills, even if you get lost sometimes!

The Motivation Corner

It's okay if the words "challenge" or "learn" make you sweat a little. Remember that the more you work, the more your brain grows! Don't worry that you're not smart enough or that it's too late. You have an extra edge because you're fasting, which gives your brain what it needs: new situations. This isn't about being perfect; it's about being open-minded, fun, and determined to help your amazing brain do its best!

Introducing Fasting: A Possible Way to Keep Your Brain Healthy and Rejuvenated

So far, we've talked about how our brains change as we age and how they can change so quickly. Finally, let's talk about an idea that might seem a little strange at first: not eating can be very good for your brain if you practice it.

Listen up, because we're about to dive into the fascinating world of fasting and how it can help you keep your brain healthy for life.

Fasting: An Old Practice and a New Science

People have been fasting for hundreds of years for a wide range of reasons, including religious, spiritual, or health-related ones. It wasn't until recently that modern science caught up and found out some really interesting things about how fasting affects the brain and the body.

Ill bust a big myth: fasting is not the same as going without food. Starvation is when you don't eat for a long time and can't stop. It is bad for your body. If you want to fast, on the other hand, you decide how much food you eat for certain amounts of time. You can think of it as giving your body a planned break from processing all the time.

What changes in the brain when you fast?

Things get really interesting now. When we don't eat for a while, our bodies stop using glucose (sugar) from food as fuel and start breaking down extra fat. This change in metabolism sets off a chain of good changes at the cellular level. These changes seem to have the biggest effect on the brain. Here are some of the most important ways that fasting might make your brain work better:

• Protection Mode: ON: Research shows that fasting may help protect brain cells from damage, which could keep them from getting worse with age as is common in Alzheimer's and Parkinson's diseases. Putting this on your brain cells is like protecting them with armor!

• Revitalization Station: Remember how we talked about autophagy, the process that cleans up cells? Autophagy works very well when you fast. This means getting rid of cell waste and other things that can clog things up. This could improve the health and efficiency of brain cells.

• Mental Growth Spurt: It has been shown that fasting raises amounts of BDNF, a special protein that helps brain cells grow and stay healthy. It also improves memory and learning.

More than just buzzwords: What Does This Mean for You?

While the science is interesting, what does it mean in the real world? Researchers and people who fast often say that it has perks like

• Clearer Thinking: Picture those foggy days going away and being replaced by days when your mind is more clear and focused. When you use Memory Power-Up, you'll have fewer frustrating "it's on the tip of my tongue" moments and be able to remember names, times, and other useful information.

• Mood Booster: Fasting may improve your mood and help lower your worry, which can make you feel calm and mentally healthy. There is no one-size-fits-all way to fast.

It's important to note that fasting can be done in different ways. We will talk more about the different choices, such as intermittent fasting and longer, controlled fasts, in the next chapters.

We will also talk about how to find the best option for you as you age. For now, the most important thing to remember is that fasting is not a way to severely limit what you eat. Instead, it's about using your body's natural ability to heal and rejuvenate in a smart way, and your brain is ready to get really good results.

Something to cheer you up

It's okay if the thought of fasting makes you feel uncomfortable or new. Think of this as the start of an adventure. You are about to learn how fasting can be a useful, easy to do, and safe tool. The best thing? You get to try out the possible brain-boosting effects for yourself! It's not enough to just read reports; you have to choose to take care of your amazing brain for the long term.

Let me know if you'd like to talk about any other possible benefits of fasting or add any other motivating factors. I can't wait to keep working on this book with you!

Chapter 2: The Power of Fasting: Beyond Weight Loss

Okay, so now you're interested in how fasting might help your brain. But let's be clear on what fasting really means before we talk about the different ways to do it.

Don't believe what you think you know about crash diets and going without food. You're not being punished when you fast; it's a powerful way to give your body (and, as we'll see, your brain!) a chance to reset and heal. This is what's going on:

How Fasting Works: It's Not Just Skipping Meals

For the most part, fasting means not eating any food for a set amount of time. It's about giving your digestive system a break so that your body can focus on other important tasks, like getting rid of trash and fixing cells.

The main difference between fasting and hungry is that starving is a state of not being able to eat. On the other hand, fasting is a choice you make to give your body a break from constantly digesting food.

Fasting has been done for a long time; it's not a trend.

People of many faiths and cultures have been fasting for hundreds of years. It wasn't just for religious reasons; people knew in their hearts that resting their bodies was good for them.

Now, science is catching up and showing us the interesting ways that fasting affects our health, including our brainpower!

How to Find Your Fit: The Many Faces of Fasting

It's great that fasting can be done in different ways. You can't use the same method for everyone. Below is a list of some common ways you can try:

1. Time-Restricted Eating (TRE): This method is all about limiting the amount of time you can eat each day. Imagine ending your dinner at 8 p.m., not eating breakfast, and then not eating again until noon the next day. This makes a 16-hour fasting window every day (hello, 16:8 method!). TRE is a great way to ease into fasting, and it's easy to fit into most people's lives.

2. When you follow the 5:2 diet, you eat normally for five days out of the week. For the last two days, you limit your calories to between 500 and 600, but not in a row. It's a good choice for people who like an organized but flexible approach.

3. A 24-hour fast is part of the Eat Stop Eat method once or twice a week. Since it's a more intense method, you should talk to your doctor before starting. On the other hand, some people like how simple a once-a-week fast is.

4. Alternate-Day Fasting (ADF): With this method, you eat normally some days and too few calories (about 500 calories) on other days. Even though it can be hard, the rhythm of switching days can work well for some people.

Note: Pay attention to your body at all times! If you've never fasted before, start slowly and slowly make your fasting time longer. During your fast, it's also important to drink plenty of water. Of course, if you already have any health problems, you should talk to your doctor before starting any fasting journey.

Beyond the Basics: Things to Think About for People Over 40

When you get to be at least 40 years old, there are some extra things you should think about when you are thinking about fasting:

• Medicines: During a fast, some medicines may need to be changed. Talk to your doctor for advice.

• Managing Blood Sugar: If you have diabetes or are at risk for diabetes, you need to plan your fasting carefully to keep your blood sugar levels healthy.

Hydration is Key: This is important for everyone, but it's even more important as we get older. During your fast, make sure you drink plenty of water.

Don't get too confused by all the choices!

What's good? To fast, there is no one "right" way. The important thing is to find a way that works for you and your lifestyle. Here are some ways to do things. Think of them as a menu. Take what works for you.

This is the real payoff of fasting: you lose more than just weight. We already said that fasting isn't just for losing weight. Finally, some study shows that fasting may have many health benefits, these being some of them:

• Better brainpower: As we've already talked about, fasting can be like a mental spring cleaning, which could improve memory, focus, and general brain function. You'll feel better after this.

• Cellular Renewal: Do you remember autophagy, the process by which cells are recycled? It speeds up when you fast, which might make your body (and brain!) healthy and stronger.

• Preventing Disease: Some studies show that fasting may help lower the chance of getting long-term diseases like diabetes, heart disease, and even some types of cancer. It could be a very useful tool for keeping your body in good shape.

Important: Fasting won't solve all your problems. This tool works best when used along with good habits like eating well, working out, and dealing with stress. It's like the magic ingredient that makes everything you do work better.

Changing Your Mindset: Taking on the Challenge

At first, the thought of not eating might seem scary. But here's the deal: facing challenges is how you strengthen your mind (because, let's face it, your brain needs exercise just like your body!).

Remember the first time you did any kind of exercise. Did you feel at ease right away? Most likely not. But as you kept going, it got easier, and you started to see results. In the same way, fasting works. Those initial hunger pangs will go away, and as you start to feel better mentally and your health might get better, you'll start to see these rare fasts as empowering, not depriving.

A Word About Safety

Most healthy people can safely fast as long as they follow some common-sense rules. But some people, especially those with any of the following conditions, might need more careful help:

• Being pregnant or breastfeeding

• Having diabetes

• a history of eating problems

• A few basic health problems

Always talk to your doctor to figure out what you need and make a plan that works for you.

Take a break when your body tells you to.

As you start to fast, keep these signs in mind to know when it's time to break your fast and eat:

• Feeling lightheaded or dizzy

• Strong, constant hunger

• Severe shaking or confusion

You haven't failed! Instead, it's your body telling you it needs food. You can always try again another day, maybe when you have less time to fast.

The experiment starts!

You will be in charge of your own fasting journey from now on. We'll talk more about the different types of fasting, how to ease into them, and how to get the most out of the possible brain-boosting effects in the next few chapters. Accept that you are curious, pay attention to how you react, and let the findings drive you.

This chapter talks about the history of fasting and how it has been used for thousands of years.

Fasting might seem like just another health trend when we think about it. For thousands of years, though, people have known that fasting can help them, even before there were science studies to back it up. Let's look into its interesting history:

Spiritual Traditions: Bringing the Soul and Body Together

Different kinds of fasting are a part of many major religions, such as Christianity, Judaism, Islam, Buddhism, and Hinduism. People didn't just fast to clean their bodies; they saw it as a powerful spiritual practice that could help them become more self-disciplined, connect with God more deeply, and get clear on their innermost thoughts.

Fasting as Medicine by Ancient Healers

Did you know that Hippocrates, who is known as the "father of modern medicine," believed that fasting could help people get better? Medical professionals in ancient Greece, Rome, and China thought that resting the digestive system could help the body heal itself faster. They were pretty close!

Through the Ages: A Way to Stay Strong

When there wasn't enough food, people had to fast. People from all over the world have, however, chosen to fast at different times throughout history, even when food was plentiful. This shows that they had a natural sense of the possible benefits that went beyond just watching their calories.

Now we're in modern science.

Even though the idea of fasting may seem old, scientists have only recently started to look into how it affects health. The new results, on the other hand, are very exciting:

• Cellular Superstars: New research helps us understand why fasting seems to be good for the brain and body. Researchers have found ideas like autophagy (recycling of cells) and BDNF production (growth of brain cells) that explain how those old observations came to be.

• Powerhouse for preventing disease: Studies are starting to show a link between fasting and possible changes in insulin resistance, blood sugar control, and a decrease in inflammation. All of these are important for fighting chronic diseases.

• The Brain Boost: Exciting study about how fasting might help protect our brains from age-related decline and improve cognitive function has been in the news. For those of us over 40, this is where it really hits home!

Old habits and new knowledge are linked in an interesting way. It's amazing how many of the views people held in the past are now being supported by modern science. As it turns out, those spiritual fasts and traditional healing methods may have helped a lot more than just the body. They may have also benefited cells and the brain in ways we're just now starting to understand.

Lessons We Can Learn from Our Past

What can we learn about fasting from all of this history?

• Be respectful of the tradition: fasting isn't a new trend. Knowing its deep past can give us more drive and a sense that we are connected to something much bigger than ourselves.

• Have faith in your body's natural abilities: People have lived and thrived during times of plenty and lack. Our bodies are amazingly strong and can use natural ways to heal themselves when they get the chance.

• More Than Willpower: Self-discipline is important, but fasting can teach us to pay more attention to and value our bodies' signals.

Science Backs Up the Wisdom

The great thing is that we don't have to only look at things from the past for ideas. Modern science has given us the chance to learn the interesting "why" behind the possible benefits of fasting.

Using both old wisdom and cutting-edge study together is a powerful way to get things done.

You are a part of the change

It's an important step in your health journey to look into fasting as a way to improve your brain health and general health. You could see yourself as both following an old practice and trying new things with your own body.

Use history to fuel your drive.

When you know about the background of fasting, you can approach it with more than just a weight-loss mindset. Think of yourself as tapping into a source of ancient knowledge that is backed up by exciting new findings. This will allow your body to reach its full potential for healing and rejuvenation.

Key Mechanisms That Fasting Is Good for the Brain

Imagine that your brain is a busy city with millions of people who work hard every day. Fasting can be thought of as a planned project to improve the city by getting rid of the old and making room for the new. This makes the whole system work better.

Here is a list of some of the interesting processes at work:

Mechanism #1: Autophagy, which is your brain's cleaning crew

Think of tiny robots that recycle moving through your brain cells. That's basically autophagy. It's a normal process by which cells get rid of damaged or worn-out parts and recycle them. Misfolded proteins are linked to brain diseases.

It's important because autophagy slows down with age, which can cause a growth of cell junk. When you fast, autophagy speeds up. This cleans out your brain and may lower your risk of cognitive loss that comes with getting older.

Mechanism #2: BDNF Boost—Building a Brain That Does Well

Bear in mind BDNF? This amazing protein feeds your brain, encouraging the growth of new cells, strengthening links, and building up your memory and ability to learn.

• What it means: It has been shown that fasting raises BDNF levels. No matter what age you are, having more BDNF in your brain can help it stay smart, flexible, and strong.

Mechanism #3: Reducing stress and calming the internal storm

The stress hormone cortisol floods your brain when you're under a lot of worry. This is terrible for your memory, attention, and mood over time.

Why it matters: Fasting helps keep cortisol levels in check and may raise production of the "feel-good" chemical GABA, which makes you feel calm and makes your brain better able to handle stress.

Mechanism #4: Ketone Power: An Alternative Fuel Source for Your Brain

When you fast, your body stops using glucose (sugar) as fuel and starts burning fat stores instead, which makes ketone bodies. Ketones do more than just fuel your body; they also seem to be good for your brain.

• Why It Matters: Studies show that ketones may help protect brain cells, lower inflammation, and make your brain make more energy. Some studies show that ketones can help your brain work better and keep you from some brain diseases that come with getting older.

Mechanism #5: Lowering Inflammation - Putting out the fire in your brain

A lot of health problems, from heart disease to sadness, are caused by low-grade inflammation that lasts for a long time. Did you know that your brain can be hurt? Aging makes it harder to think clearly and remember things.

• Why It Matters: Research shows that fasting may help reduce inflammation in the brain and body. Less inflammation can help you think more clearly, feel better, and maybe even lower your risk of getting brain disease.

The Whole Story: A New Brain

It's not just one of these processes working by itself; it's how they all work together that's really powerful. When you fast, it's like setting off a chain of good things for your brain:

• Spring Cleaning and New Construction: You're getting rid of waste (autophagy) and building better brain structures at the same time (BDNF boost).

• Zen Master Mode: By lowering stress and inflammation, fasting can help you feel calm, focused, and have a clearer mind.

• Powerhouse of adaptability: As you age, your brain's metabolism becomes more flexible, making it easier to switch between food sources. It may also become more resistant to changes that come with getting older.

What Could This Mean for You in the Real World?

It's cool that science is exciting, but let's get real:

• "Zip Up That Brain Fog": Picture days when your brain fog goes away, leaving you with better clarity and focus in its place.

• Improve Memory: You'll have fewer annoying "it's on the tip of my tongue" moments and be able to remember important things more easily.

• Take on the Challenge: It's easy to learn, it can spark new interests, and it keeps your brain active and sharp.

• Emotional Superhero: Feeling stronger, better able to control your mood, and able to deal with life's stresses without getting stressed.

The Motivation Corner

Remember that your brain is not fixed; you can definitely change how healthy it is! Fasting gives your brain a lot of strong tools that can help it work better. Would you like to speed up the process of repair, renewal, and growth? Because that's the kind of chance you're looking for.

Dispelling Myths and Getting Used to the Idea of Fasting

The word "fasting" can make us worry and think the wrong things. Let's face some of the most common ones head-on and get rid of fear and doubt by giving people information and a sense of power.

Myth No. 1: Going without Food Is Fasting.

Certainly not! Remember that fasting is a choice that you make, not a state of random lack like starvation. By following fasting plans, you give your brain and body a break from the steady cycle of digestion while still making sure you get enough food and water.

Myth #2: If I fast, my metabolism will slow down.

This is a big one that's not true at all! If you fast for a short time, your metabolism may speed up a little. But even if there is a small drop, it's generally only temporary and not very big. The deal is that when you don't eat as much, your body burns stored energy more efficiently. This is because your metabolism changes to use your fat stores as energy.

Myth #3: If you fast for a long time, you'll lose muscle.

People who are athletes or very busy should be most worried about this myth. Some muscle loss can happen during a very long fast (which we won't be doing!), but the kind of moderate, time-limited fasts we'll talk about actually help your body use saved energy for fuel more efficiently and can help you keep your lean muscle mass if done correctly.

Myth #4: Fasting will make you weak and hungry.

Okay, there is some truth to this, especially at the beginning! You should expect that initial stage of getting used to not snacking all the time. You may feel a little more hungry, a little more irritable, and a little more tired for a short time. The great news? As your body gets used to the changes, these feelings generally go away in a few days.

Myth #5: It's bad to fast.

Adults who are generally healthy can safely fast for short periods of time as long as they follow the right rules. But it's very important to talk to your doctor first, especially if you are on any medications or have any health problems. They can help you make sure that fasting fits your goals and not against them.

Remember that it's important to pay attention to your body! You should start slowly and slowly lengthen your fasts. If you feel sick, dizzy, or very faint for a long time, break your fast and try again another time, maybe with a shorter window!

Easing in: The Way to Gain Power

Fasting is a lot like starting a new workout plan. After years of sitting on the couch, you wouldn't try to run a race, right? Let's break down a step-by-step plan that is easy to follow:

• Step 1: Make the overnight stretch longer. Are you not eating between dinner and breakfast already? First, try to go without food for 12 hours straight. Gradually extend this time to fast to 14 to 16 hours a few times a week.

• Step 2: Try Time-Restricted Eating (TRE). Once you're used to the longer overnight fasts, look into TRE plans like the 16:8 way. This means that you should eat all of your meals within an 8-hour window and not eat for 16 hours.

• Step 3: Think about longer fasts (optional): If TRE feels good and you want to take things a step further, talk to your doctor about whether or not it is safe to add rare 24-hour fasts to your plan. How to Make the Change Go More Easily:

• Step 4: Hydration is key: drink a lot of water during your fasting times to help with headaches and hunger.

• Step 5: Do you really feel hungry (growling stomach, etc.)? Listen to True Hunger. Or is it habit or boredom? Try something fun, like going for a walk or writing in a book.

• Step 6: Choose what you eat: When you break your fast, eat whole, unprocessed foods, protein, and healthy fats to keep you full and energetic.

How You Think Is Everything!

Try fasting as an experiment in taking better care of yourself. Pay attention to how your mind and body react. The full benefits won't show up right away, so enjoy the small wins along the way, like having more energy, a clearer mind, and a stronger sense of control.

Do not forget that fasting is not a punishment but a tool. Accept it as a new way to take care of your wonderful brain and help it reach its full potential!

Chapter 3: Intermittent Fasting: Flexible and Effective

Some types of intermittent fasting are time-restricted eating, fasting every other day, and so on.

Intermittent fasting is great because there is no one right way to do it. Let's take a look at some of the most popular and easy-to-use IF techniques and talk about what they do and who they might work best for:

Type 1: Time-Restricted Eating (TRE): This is the best tool for beginners.

• What It Is: TRE means eating all of your meals during a certain time frame every day and then not eating for the rest of the time. For many people, the 16:8 way works best. This plan involves fasting for 16 hours and then eating for 8 hours. If you're just starting to fast, you can also try a 14:10 or even a 12:12.

• Why It's Awesome: TRE is a method that's pretty easy for beginners to understand. You probably already fast overnight; TRE just makes the fasting last a little longer. Most people can easily fit it into their plans.

• Who It's Great For: People who are new to fasting, don't like rules that are too strict, and want to make a long-term change to their lifestyle that will improve their brain function and general health.

Type 2: Alternate-Day Fasting (ADF): Taking It to the Next Level

What It Is: ADF involves going back and forth between "feast" days, when you eat normally, and "fast" days, when you either eat very few calories (usually around 500) or don't eat at all for 24 hours. Why it's great: Research shows that ADF may have some big metabolic benefits and may help you lose weight. For some, it's easy to stick to the simple rule of switching days.

• Who It's Great For: People who are ready for a more difficult method and people who want to see if they can speed up their metabolism. It is important to remember that ADF might not work for everyone, so it is very smart to talk to your doctor before starting this method.

Type 3: The 5:2 Diet: An Option for Part-Time Fast Users

For this method to work, you eat usually five days a week and then limit your calories to 500 to 600 for two days in a row.

• What makes it great: The 5:2 diet gives you options while still including those stricter, possibly metabolism-boosting fast days. It might work well for people who like order but don't want to fast all the time.

• It's great for people who like to stick to a plan, have trouble with longer fasts, or who like the idea of fasting only twice a week. **Type 4: The Warrior Diet: For People Who Like to Do Extreme Experiments**

• What It Is: This strict method includes a 20-hour fast every day and a 4-hour "feast" window in the evening. It tells you to eat mostly whole foods during the feeding time.

• What makes it great: The Warrior Diet may cause you to cut back on calories a lot, but the short time you have to eat makes sure you get enough protein. For some, the strict framework is what drives them.

• Who It's Good For: This method is NOT good for people who are just starting out. It's better for experienced fasters, people who can carefully plan a 4-hour meal that's high in nutrients, and people who want to take on a bigger task.

Bonus: Longer fasts every so often: Going deeper (with care)

Fasts that last at least 48 hours can have extra benefits, but they also have more risks. These kinds of fasts should ONLY be done with a doctor's help, and they're not the main topic of this book. For those who want to learn more with the help of their doctor, it's still worth quickly mentioning them.

A Note on Being Flexible: Change to Fit Your Life

Don't think of intermittent fasting as a strict set of rules. Here's how to make it work for you, especially as you get older:

• Change When You Eat: The cool thing about TRE is that you can change when you eat and when you fast every day. Work obligations or plans with friends? Change as needed!

• Pay attention to your body: There are days when a 16-hour fast is easy and days when 12 hours feels better. Follow your body's cues!

• Aim for progress instead of perfection: It's okay to miss a fast or shorten your time once in a while. Making sure you do it every time is key!

The Motivation Corner

View this as an exciting adventure! You can try different types of fasting to find the one that works best for your body, your tastes, and your way of life. By giving your body these planned breaks, you're letting its amazing ability to heal itself shine through, especially in your brain!

How to Get Started with Intermittent Fasting

You don't have to go into complete deprivation when you start intermittent fasting. A personalized, step-by-step plan that helps you build energy, both physically and mentally, is the key to success. Let's make a step-by-step plan to help you find your fasting flow!

Stage 1: Warming Up—Let Your Natural Fast Last Longer

You are fasting while you sleep and don't even know it! Your first step is to slowly make that overnight fast last a little longer:

• Goal: 12 to 14 hours: Try to wait 12 to 14 hours between dinner and breakfast. Dinner is still being eaten at 8 p.m. Just change the time of breakfast to 8 or 9 am.

• Take small steps: add one hour at a time at first. Once 12 hours seems like enough time, try adding 30 minutes more. Pay attention to your body; it will tell you how fast to go.

• Pay Attention to Your Hunger: Signs of real hunger, like a growling stomach and a noticeable drop in energy, are different from the urges to snack. Keep track of how you feel as you extend the overnight fast.

Stage 2: Start eating only during certain times (TRE)

As soon as you feel good with slightly longer overnight fasts, it's time for TRE! Remember that this method is very flexible and easy for beginners:

• Choose a Plan: Start with a 14:10 or 16:8 plan. If you follow the 16:8 rule, you should go without food for 16 hours and then eat all of your meals within 8 hours.

• The Power of Being Able to Change: Every day doesn't have to be the same for when you eat. Why not skip breakfast and just eat lunch and dinner? It works great! Find a pace that works for you.

• Planning your meals (slightly) is important. You don't need complicated plans, but think about what you'll eat for your first meal after the fast. Protein and good fats will make you feel full for a longer time.

Stage 3 : Leveling up (optional)

Ready to live with TRE for a few weeks? You might be ready to try fasters that are harder, but remember that you can always choose not to!

• Welcome to Alternate-Day Fasting (ADF): Take it easy at first. One day a week should be a full fast or a 500-calorie fast. If you can handle it well, you can gradually increase the number of calories you eat.

• How the 5:2 Diet Works: Pick two days a week that don't follow each other to severely limit your calories. What you eat the other days should be normal and healthy.

• The key is self-discovery: Pay close attention to how your mind and body react to these longer fasting times. There will be people who don't like them, and that's okay. TRE is great on its own!

How to Do Well at Any Level:

• Drink lots of water, herbal teas, and black coffee. These will help you control your hunger pangs and fight headaches and tiredness, especially as your body adjusts.

• Don't Ignore Real Hunger: If you feel faint, dizzy, or very sick, eat a light snack to break your fast. You can try again tomorrow!

• Eat whole foods. When you do eat, break your fast with meals that are high in protein, healthy fats, and colorful veggies to get the most out of the benefits for your body and brain.

• Keep track of your progress: Write down how you feel before and after fasts, including how much energy you have, how clear your mind is, etc. It's important to remember that IF isn't right for everyone. These wins will keep you going when things get tough.

Before you start, you should always talk to your doctor, especially if you are already sick or on medicine.

The Change in Mindset: Getting Stronger While You Fast

There is a time of getting used to fasting, just like when you start a new workout routine. On the other hand, just like working out makes your muscles stronger, fasting makes your body and mind very flexible. So here it is:

• The first few days: The Bravest: You can expect to feel hungry and have low energy. Keep going, because these usually go away pretty quickly!

• Energy Upswing: After the first change, a lot of people say they feel more focused and clear-headed. Happy to see these wins!

• It's Not About Deprivation: Think about how empowering it is to give your brain and body a break from nonstop digestion to start those amazing processes of healing.

The Motivation Corner

Enjoy the journey! It's okay to start slowly and slowly increase the amount of time you fast as your body allows. Any fast, no matter how short, is good for your health. You will definitely find the strategies that work best for your body, brain, and way of life since there are so many to choose from.

Adapting IF to suit your life over 40: schedules and sample plans

IF is great because it's not a rigid plan that works for everyone. Flexibility is your best friend as you deal with work, family, and the unique changes that happen after age 40. Let's talk about fasting schedules, sample plans, and ways to make sure that it works with your life instead of getting in the way!

Things to Think About When you're 40 or older

When making your fasting plan, here are some things to keep in mind as you get older:

• Managing medications: Fasting might change when or how much of some drugs you should take. It is important to talk to your doctor first.

• Energy: It may take a little longer for your body to get used to fasting. Wait until you find the best time to fast, and pay attention to your body's energy signs.

• Changes in hormones (especially in women): Changes in hormones can make some women feel more hungry or cause their blood sugar to rise and fall. During your eating times, focus on foods that are high in nutrients.

Schedule Examples Getting into the Rhythm

Let's look at some ways that TRE can be used in different types of lives. Remember that these are just starting points. Make changes as needed!

Schedule 1: The Busy Professional

- Eating Window: 11am to 7pm (16:8 method)

- Benefits: Ending the fast around lunchtime allows for energy during peak work hours and enjoying an earlier dinner with family or for social plans.

Schedule 2: The Early Riser

- Eating Window: 7am to 3pm (16:8 method)

- Benefits: Fits those naturally early schedules and leaves evenings free for relaxing and earlier bedtimes (crucial for brain health!)

Schedule 3: Shift Work Friendly

- Eating Window: Adjusted daily depending on work schedule (e.g., breaking fast after your shift, then squeezing in two more meals before the next shift starts)

- Benefits: Adapts IF even with unpredictable hours. Focus on prioritizing a few hours of fasting when possible and nourishing meals during eating windows.

Sample Meal Plans: The Basics

No need for fancy meals here! Prioritize whole foods, lean protein, and plenty of vegetables for maximum brain benefits:

Post-Fast Meal 1: Energy Booster

- Scrambled eggs with spinach and avocado toast

- Greek yogurt with berries and a handful of nuts

Post-Fast Meal 2: Balanced and Satisfying

- Grilled chicken salad with mixed greens, variety of veggies, and light dressing

- Lentil soup with a whole-wheat roll

Post-Fast Meal 3: Nourishing Dinner

- Baked salmon with roasted vegetables and quinoa

- Turkey meatballs with whole-wheat pasta and marinara sauce

Smart Snacking (If Needed)

Ideally, you'll feel satisfied during fasting periods. But, if you need a boost, opt for:

- A handful of nuts

- Hard-boiled egg

- Bone broth (great source of electrolytes)

- Small piece of fruit

Adapting for Longer Fasts (With Caution)

If you opt for ADF or the 5:2 Diet, here's how to adjust:

• ADF "Feast Day" Tips: Focus on whole foods and prioritize good hydration on these days. Don't view them as unrestricted eating binges, as you'll likely feel less than great later!

• 5:2 "Fast Day" Tips: Plan a small, nutrient-rich meal (300-500 calories) like a veggie-packed soup or salad with grilled fish. Spread a few snacks throughout the day if needed.

The Importance of Flexibility

Life happens! Here's how to handle those inevitable curveballs:

• Social Events: Don't panic! Adjust your eating window slightly, enjoy the event, and get back to your regular fasting routine the next day.

• Unexpected Hunger: Break your fast with a light snack. It's better to listen to your body than endure misery. You can always try for a longer fasting window next time.

• Travel Time: Take advantage of long flights or car rides as built-in fasts. Pack healthy snacks in case your ideal eating window isn't possible.

The Motivation Corner

Remember that fasting for any length of time may be good for you! Don't let trying to be perfect get in the way of your progress. This is what will really make a difference for your brain and health in the long run, even if you only fast for a short time. Enjoy every step that fits into your busy life after 40!

Chapter 4: Extended Fasting Options

Exploring Longer Fasts (24 Hours +)

So far, we've talked about ways to do intermittent fasting that are easy to fit into your daily life. But what if you want to fast for longer than those small periods of time?

Longer fasts, usually 24 hours or more, might make some of the benefits we've already talked about even stronger. They do, however, come with more risks and aren't right for everyone.

Important: If you are taking medicine or already have a health problem, you should only go on a long-term fast with the help of a trained medical professional. This section is just for your knowledge; it's not meant to replace medical advice!

Why Should You Think About Longer Fasts?

Here are some of the possible benefits of these longer fasts that make people want to try them:

• Faster Autophagy: When you fast for longer amounts of time, your body speeds up autophagy, which is a great process for cleaning out cells. This might help get rid of the dead cells and other junk that makes you age and causes diseases related to getting older.

• Deeper Metabolic Reset: Some studies show that longer fasts may cause a more major metabolic shift, making your body better at using fat as fuel and making insulin work more efficiently.

• Better mental clarity: Many people say that long fasts help them focus and think clearly. This may be because long fasts cause your brain to make ketones, which are its alternative fuel source.

• Possible Protection Against Disease: More research needs to be done, but early studies suggest that longer fasts may help lower the chance of some chronic diseases and make people live longer.

Being aware of the risks

Long-term fasts need to be carefully thought out. Here are some bad things that might happen:

• Not for Everyone: People with diabetes, eating disorders, who are pregnant or breastfeeding, or who have other health problems should NOT try long fasting without close medical supervision.

• Nutrient Deficiencies: If you don't plan ahead, long fasts can leave you short on nutrients. It's important to talk to your doctor about supplements.

• Possible Side Effects: Headaches, tiredness, anger, and trouble focusing are all possible, especially on the first try.

• Harder to Keep Up: Both physically and mentally, it can be much harder to keep up with longer fasts.

Different kinds of long fasts

If you want to find out more before talking to your doctor, here is a quick list of some common ways to do it:

• Fasting for 24 to 36 hours is a good way to start fasting for longer amounts of time. Do this once or twice a week.

• Multi-Day Water Fasts: People who do these fasts only drink water for two to three days, or sometimes longer. There are more risks with this method because it is more extreme.

• FMDs, or fasting-like diets: A 5-day very low-calorie diet is part of this method, which is usually overseen by a doctor. It is meant to have the same benefits as fasting while giving you some nutrients.

How to Make Extended Fasting Safer (While Being Supervised by a Doctor!)

If your doctor says it's okay, here are some things you can do to improve your chances:

• Go Slowly: Don't start a multi-day fast right away! Start with shorter IF and one-day fasts and work your way up to see how your body responds.

• Drink plenty of water. Electrolyte problems can happen during long fasts. If your doctor tells you to, you might want to take electrolyte pills along with drinking enough water.

• Watch Out for Low Energy: During long fasts, don't do intense exercise or drive long distances. If your body tells you it needs to rest, do it.

• Take it easy: It takes skill to break a long fast. To keep your digestive system from getting too stressed, start with light broths and then eat small meals that are easy to digest.

The Motivation Corner

Long-term fasts have a lot of promise, but they're not a magic bullet. Remember that even the short-term irregular fasts we talked about have great effects, such as improving metabolic health, brain function, and autophagy. Think of them as strong tools you use every day to improve your health over time.

Why individualization is important

There is no race in fasting! It's up to you to find the best way to fast. Respect your body and what it needs, whether you stick to 16:8 TRE or go on a planned longer fast once in a while.

You don't have to go too far; you just need to find the right rhythm to get the amazing benefits of fasting in a safe and healthy way.

Safety Tips and When to See a Doctor

Even though fasting can be very good for your health and brain function, it doesn't mean you can ignore your body's needs. An important part of fasting, especially for people over 40, is knowing when to talk to your doctor and what warning signs to look out for.

Before fasting, you should definitely talk to your doctor if you have:

• Diabetes (Type 1 or Type 2): Fasting can have a big effect on blood sugar levels, so it's important to carefully handle medications and stay under medical supervision.

• A history of eating disorders: People who have or have had eating disorders in the past may find fasting difficult. For a safe and supported method, it's important to get help.

If you are pregnant or breastfeeding, you shouldn't fast because your body needs food more than anything else.

• Long-Term Health Problems: These include kidney or liver disease, heart problems, thyroid problems, or any other serious health problem. Your doctor needs to make sure that fasting fits in with the way you are being treated.

• Dependence on Medicines: A lot of medicines need to be taken with food or with different amounts of water during fasting periods. Don't change the way you take your medicine without first talking to your doctor.

Signs of trouble: Stop fasting and see a doctor if you have any of these symptoms:

• Severe dizziness or fainting: This could mean that your blood pressure is too low or that your electrolytes are out of balance.

• Heart palpitations or an irregular heartbeat: It's important to make sure that you don't have any heart problems that are getting worse because you're fasting.

• Feeling sick or throwing up all the time: This could mean you're dehydrated or having a bad reaction that needs medical help.

• Extreme Weakness or Confusion: These symptoms need to be carefully looked at because they could be caused by changes in blood sugar or other problems.

• Fainting: If you lose awareness, you need to see a doctor right away. Don't brush this off!

What You Need to Know, Even If You're Usually Healthy

Before beginning a new diet or way of life, especially one that involves fasting, it's always a good idea to have a quick talk with your doctor. These professionals can give you specific help and make sure that this strong tool is safe to use with your general health.

Extra Things to Think About When you're 40 or older

Our bodies change on their own as we age. Even though fasting can still be very helpful, here are some things to remember:

• Carefully check your blood sugar: Insulin sensitivity can change with age, even if you don't have diabetes. If you feel shaky or off, check your blood sugar.

• Put electrolytes first: As we get older, it's even more important to stay hydrated and maybe take extra electrolytes during fasts.

Longer fasts might not be as dangerous: For many people, short fasts are better for them and pose less of a risk than longer fasting times. Pay attention to your body at all times!

How Doctor and Faster Work Together

Your healthcare team should be seen as your fasting friends. For those who want to try longer fasts, it is important to have ongoing help and monitoring from a knowledgeable doctor. Among these are:

• Bloodwork at the start: Before you fast, it can help to get a clear picture of how your blood sugar, fluids, kidneys, and liver are working.

• Regular Check-Ins: If you're fasting for a long time, your doctor may suggest that you be checked on more often to catch any problems early.

• Medication Changes: They can give you expert advice on when to take certain medicines or how much to take.

The Motivation Corner

Putting safety first isn't a sign of weakness; it means you care about your health! You care about your body and want to use fasting in a way that gives you the most benefits with the least amount of risk by choosing to talk to your doctor.

Remember that even if you only fast for a short time, your body will still get huge benefits from it in terms of brain and cell health. You can change how you fast, and working with your doctor will help you find the best way to do it that is safe, sustainable, and very powerful!

Gradual Ways to Do Longer Fasts

Getting ready for a longer fast is a lot like getting ready for a run. You wouldn't think you could run 26.2 miles on your first try, would you? The same is true for fasting: slowly building up your "endurance" lets your body adapt, which raises your chances emotionally and physically.

A very important thing to keep in mind is that consistent intermittent fasting is very helpful, even if longer fasts are your end goal. With much shorter fasting times, you can get that daily cellular renewal and possible brain power boost.

Stage 1: Get good at intermittent fasting

Before going into longer periods of fasting, you need to get good at time-restricted eating (TRE):

• The goal of 16:8: Aim to go without food for 16 hours straight and eat every 8 hours for a few weeks or even months.

• Play around and make adjustments: Figure out the best time to eat based on your plan and how hungry you are. Try overnight fasts that are a little longer or a little shorter to find your best pace.

• Focus on Whole Foods: To get the most out of the benefits, feed your body whole, unprocessed foods, protein, healthy fats, and colorful veggies during eating windows.

Stage 2: Telling people about the 24-hour fast

If you're good at your TRE program, you can start experimenting with extended fasting:

• Be Smart About Your Day: You should pick a day when you don't have to do a lot of work or hard exercise.

• Make plans for the break: Pick a short, healthy meal to eat to break your fast. You could have bone broth, veggie soup, or a small amount of grilled fish and vegetables.

• Staying hydrated: During the fast, drink a lot of water and maybe take potassium supplements (talk to your doctor about this).

Stage 3: Getting better (Be Careful)

If you can handle fasting for 24 hours, you might try slightly longer windows with care:

• The 36-Hour Choice: Try doing one 36-hour fast a week, or even less often if you can. Most of the time, this means missing breakfast, lunch, and dinner one day.

• Pay close attention to your body: Are you having trouble with severe hunger pangs, extreme weakness, or mood swings? Longer fasts might not be for you. That's not a bad thing!

• Take it easy: Break up longer fasts with foods that are easy for your body to digest. Gradually increase the size of your portions to keep your digestive system from getting too full.

How to Do Well at Every Level

• Mind Over Matter: Half the fight is won when you mentally get ready for longer fasts. Think about what would happen if you succeed and tell yourself why you're doing this. Take on the task!

• An easy distraction is good for you: Keep your mind off of your hunger pangs by writing in a notebook, doing light exercise, working on a hobby project, or taking a bath.

A lot of people find it helpful to plan long fasts around days off, since sleep is a great "distractor" of hunger.

• Celebrate the Wins: Every long fast that goes well should be seen as a big win! This makes you feel more in charge and gives you more confidence.

The Motivation Corner

Don't forget that growth is better than perfection in the long run. For some, longer fasts are best, while for others, shorter daily fasts are all they need to feel better. Pay attention to your body, and don't give up if fasting for more than one day doesn't work for you. The goal is to find a rhythm that you can keep up.

Longer fasts can give you unique information about how strong your body is. They're important, but they shouldn't take over your life. You can think of them as tools you can use once in a while, until shorter fasts become a healthy habit you do every day.

Always Remember: Before going on a long fast, talk to your doctor about your specific needs and risks. With this information, you can make the right decisions to improve the health of your brain and your general well-being!

Chapter 5: Beyond Counting Hours

Fasting-Mimicking Diets: Getting Benefits Without a Full Fast

When you fast, your brain and body can work better in many ways, which we've talked about. Longer fasts, on the other hand, can be hard to keep up, and for some people, they come with more risks. Enter the fascinating world of FMDs, or diets that make you feel like you're fasting.

What Does an FMD Really Mean?

A fasting-mimicking diet is a special, usually 5-day, low-calorie, low-protein eating plan that is carefully made to make your body think it's fasting while still giving it the nutrients it needs.

In short, this is how an FMD works:

• Calorie Restriction: For a set amount of time, an FMD generally limits your daily calories to between 750 and 1100.

• Macro Magic: They focus on healthy fats and not as much on protein and carbs. This particular ratio of macronutrients is very important for getting those fasting-like effects.

• There's no free-for-all: To make sure there is a good mix of nutrients and to keep people from eating too much, most FMDs include pre-packaged meals and snacks.

• More than often under supervision: There are do-it-yourself forms of FMDs, but for your safety, especially if you already have health problems, you should talk to your doctor about this choice and maybe look into guided FMD programs.

The Possible Pros—Backed by Science

That being said, why go through all this trouble when you could just fast? FMDs have some unique benefits that could be helpful:

• Accessibility: An FMD that is properly planned is easier for many people to stick to than a water-only fast. Not having to completely give up food can be very good for your mental health.

• Safer for Some: Because FMDs contain some nutrients, they may be safer for people with certain health problems or who often don't get enough nutrients. (But always talk to your doctor!)

• Metabolic Flip: Studies show that fasting-like diets (FMDs) can cause metabolic changes similar to fasting. This could help control blood sugar, help you lose weight, and clean up your cells.

• Early research looks good: More long-term studies on humans are needed, but research suggests that FMD might help reduce inflammation, help people control their weight, and maybe even change signs related to aging.

Different kinds of FMDs

The ProLon® program, created by Dr. Valter Longo at the USC Longevity Institute, is the most well-known and researched FMD right now. Take a quick look at this:

• The Plan for ProLon®: This 5-day FMD plan comes with plant-based meals, snacks, and vitamins that are already prepared. It's meant to be done a few times a year, and healthcare workers often watch over it.

• Do-It-Yourself Methods: Some people try to copy FMD ideas by making their own low-calorie plans that focus on certain macros.

This can be harder and comes with more risks, especially when it comes to keeping the right mix of nutrients.

Important Things to Think About

Before we all join the FMD crowd, let's be honest:

Prices: Paid FMD tools like ProLon® can be pricey. Doing things yourself is cheaper, but it's also risky if you don't plan carefully.

• Not for Everyone: People with certain health problems, women who are pregnant or breastfeeding, and people who have eating disorders should not do FMDs or traditional fasts.

• Possible Side Effects: During an FMD period, some people feel tired, get headaches, or have stomach problems. Most of the time, these are brief.

• Long-Term Effects: Research on FMDs is still in its early stages, but it looks like it will be very useful. We need to do more research to fully understand the risks and benefits in the long run.

The Motivation Corner

FMDs are an interesting different way to get the same health benefits as fasting, which might make them more accessible to more people. Just think of it as another health tool you can use! Would you like to try an FMD?

So here it is: It's not always possible to use FMDs to help people. Here's how to tell if they're worth getting to know:

• You MUST get permission from a doctor: It is very important to talk to your doctor about the possible risks and benefits of an FMD, especially if you have any health issues.

• Short Fasts Feel Impossible: If the thought of a 24-hour fast makes you sweat, an FMD might be a better way to start.

• You like structure and science: FMDs, especially programs like ProLon®, offer a structured, science-based method that some people may like.

Don't forget that even short fasts can be very helpful! Find a fasting schedule that you can stick to and that puts your health and safety first in the long run.

Ketogenic diets and brain health: what they might do and what to think about Part 5: More Than Just Keeping Track of Time Most likely, you've heard of the "keto" plan. People often follow this very high-fat, very low-carbohydrate eating plan to lose weight, but it has also been shown to be good for brain health.

Let's talk about what keto is, what it might do for you, and why it's important to be careful and think about the long run.

Changes to Your Body's Fuel Source (Keto 101)

Usually, glucose (sugar) from carbs is what your body uses to power itself. But on a ketogenic diet, you eat a lot less carbs, which forces your body to find another way to get energy:

• The New Fuel Is Fat: When your body doesn't have enough glucose, it starts turning stored fat into molecules known as ketones.

• Get into ketosis: When the amount of ketones in your blood rises enough, your metabolism changes into a state called ketosis. It's like your body getting really good at burning fat for energy, both mentally and physically.

More than just losing weight, this could be good for your brain. Even though more study needs to be done, here's why keto is making people excited about the brain:

• People with epilepsy, especially kids who don't react to medicine, have used keto for decades as a way to treat their condition and help them avoid seizures.

• Neuroprotection: Some studies show that ketones might help keep brain cells from getting damaged by Alzheimer's and Parkinson's disease. But more study on people is needed.

• Clearer thinking: A lot of people say that the ketogenic diet helps them focus better, clear their minds, and maybe even keep their mood stable.

• Treating headaches: Early research suggests that a ketogenic diet might help some people decrease the number and severity of their migraines.

Note: We still don't fully understand how keto affects brain health. Long-term studies with real people are needed to fully understand the effects, including any possible risks and rewards.

Things to Think About Before You Go Keto

The ketogenic diet is a big change that needs to be carefully planned out and may need medical monitoring. Here are some things to think about:

• Dr.'s Advice Is Very Important: This is very important if you have a health problem or take medicine. Keto can change your blood sugar, cholesterol, and nutrient levels, so you should talk to a doctor before starting.

•It's not simple: Getting used to the "keto flu" (tiredness, headaches, etc.) can be hard at first. Keto also needs careful planning and tracking to make sure you get the right amount of nutrients.

• Sustainability Is Important: Is it possible to stay on a strict ketogenic diet for a long time? Adding sugar back in quickly can cancel out the benefits.

• Pay attention to whole foods: A "dirty keto" method, which means eating processed low-carb junk, doesn't get the point across. Focus on getting enough healthy fats, good protein, and veggies that aren't starchy.

• Different Persons React Differently: Just like when you fast, your body and brain react differently to keto. Some people do well, while others may have trouble. It's about trying new things on yourself!

Use keto as a tool, not as a miracle.

For some people, the ketogenic diet might be very good for their brain health. For sure, though, it won't fix everything. Think about these things:

• Mimicry of Fasting? Some experts think that the benefits of keto for the brain may come from the production of ketone bodies, which also happens when you fast.

• Is it the ketones or the lack of carbs? It needs more study to figure out how much of the benefit comes from the ketones and how much comes from cutting back on sugar and processed carbs.

• Picture of the Long Term: It's important to look into the long-term effects and safety of following a ketogenic diet, especially when it comes to brain health.

The Motivation Corner

One important thing to remember is that what you eat has a huge effect on your brain, whether you try keto or not. Cutting back on processed carbs and focusing on whole foods is good for everyone's brain. Keto may work well for some people, but it's not the only way to keep your brain healthy, smart, and strong.

Let me know if you want to talk about possible side effects or get real advice on foods that are good for you on the keto diet. We could always make smaller areas just for these details!

Customized Approaches for Finding What Works for YOU

We've talked about a lot of interesting ways that fasting can help your brain and general health. But here's the secret: there isn't just one "best" way to do things. Find what works for YOUR body, your habits, and your goals. That's the key to success.

It's important to personalize: Why a one-size-fits-all method doesn't work
Picture your body as a well-oiled machine. How you react to fasting depends on these things:

• Genes: Your genes affect everything, from how fast you enter ketosis to how your insulin levels change when you don't eat for a while.

• Health History: Long-term illnesses, medications, and how you ate and worked out in the past affect where you start and what is safe and best for you.

• Levels of stress: High levels of stress can mess up hunger hormones, which could make longer fasts harder to stick to.

• Demands of your lifestyle: Things like shift work, social obligations, and family obligations can make it hard to stick to different fasting plans.

• Personal Likes and Dislikes: Do you love breakfast or dinner early? Listen to your body's beats!

Questions to Help You Find Your Own Fasting Path

Instead of following trends without question, ask yourself these powerful questions:

• How's my wind? Pay attention to whether different lengths of fasting make you feel tired or help you think more clearly. Change your fasting dates as needed.

• Am I really hungry? Learn to tell the difference between real hunger and urges or eating habits. This helps people who are fasting not eat mindless snacks.

• What seems like it could last? If the thought of fasting for 36 hours makes you nervous, it won't work in the long run. Short fasts that are done regularly are very helpful!

• Do I like this? If fasting makes you feel bad, you need to change your plan! During eating windows, focus on eating healthy whole foods and look into ways to make fasts easier to handle.

A Guide to Customized Fasting

Are you ready to accept customization? How to do it:

• The Test on Yourself: Start with short fasts that feel good and slowly add more time. Write down how you feel and make changes based on what you see.

• Hunger Hacks: Figure out what works best for you to keep you from eating when you're hungry, like exercise, herbal tea, a creative project, etc.

• Be willing to change things: Don't be hard on yourself if you break your fast early sometimes because you have to go to a party or are sick. The next day, get back on track!

• Planning meals is important: To keep wants to a minimum during fasts, eat tasty, filling meals during eating windows.

• Keep track of your progress: Do more than just lose weight. Write down any good changes you notice, like better focus, more energy, better sleep, or anything else.

Support tailored to you: Think about hiring a professional.

If you need extra help on this journey, especially if you already have health problems, think about these options:

• A knowledgeable nutritionist can help you make a plan with the best combinations of meals to go with the way you've decided to fast.

• A health coach who knows how to fast: They can help you make changes to your attitude, deal with problems, and hold you accountable.

• A doctor who specializes in fasting: Find them if you want detailed tracking of your bloodwork and personalized advice. This is especially important if you are thinking about longer or FMD-like protocols.

The Motivation Corner

It's not going to be harder to use this personalized method; it will make things SMARTER! You can make changes that last by paying attention to your body's signs and figuring out what really works for YOU.

You don't have to fast or eat in a certain way for the longest time. It's about enjoying small wins and slow changes over time.

How Patience Can Help You Find Yourself

It takes time to find your own fasting flow. Do not rush! You learn something about your body and mind every time you fast, no matter how easy or hard it was.

You not only get healthier after each experiment, but you also learn more about yourself and feel like you have more power over your health. That really gives you power!

Chapter 6: Sharpen Your Memory

How Fasting Can Improve Memory Formation and Recall

You can think of fasting as giving your brain a memory-cleaning spring cleaning. It turns out that temporarily not eating might not seem like a good way to improve your brainpower, but it can actually cause a series of changes that make your memory better. This is how it breaks down:

Mechanism #1: Mechanism The Whole Story Is BDNF

Remember that protein BDNF that helps the brain that we talked about before? It is a big part of remembering!

• What is BDNF? Brain-Derived Neurotrophic Factor (BDNF) helps brain cells grow and stay healthy. It's like fuel for your brain cells. A brain network that has more BDNF is stronger.

• Fasting to Save the Day! Researchers have found that fasting can raise BDNF levels, which may improve the link between brain cells that help us remember things.

Mechanism #2: A Powerhouse of New Brain Cells

Prepare to geek out for a moment! A process called neurogenesis has been linked to fasting. Neurogenesis means the birth of new brain cells, especially in the hippocampus, an area important for learning and memory.

• Why it's Important: It's normal to lose some brain cells as you get older, but fasting might help your brain make more new cells to make up for that loss and keep your memory sharp.

Mechanism #3: The cleanup crew is working extra hard

We have talked about autophagy, the process by which cells recycle old parts and make room for new ones. Fasting speeds up autophagy, which is good for your brain in other ways as well:

• Get rid of the old: fasting can help get rid of misfolded proteins and cell waste that can make it hard to remember things and think clearly in general. It's kind of like getting rid of brain fog.

• Keeping the Memory Vault safe: Alzheimer's and other diseases that destroy memories may be less likely to happen if brain cells are protected from damage that comes with getting older.

What Could This Mean for You in the Real World?

Not as much of this: "What was his name again?" "Where on earth did I put my glasses?" and this more:

• Hi, Remember! You may find it easier to remember important names or details from a recent chat.

• Mental Sharpness: You'll be able to concentrate better, which will make studying or picking up a new skill easier and more fun.

• Keeping your memories safe: You can rest easy knowing that you're doing something to keep those special memories safe as you get older.

Science Spotlight: New Findings on Fasting and Memory

A lot of the study has been done on animals, but the results look good! Here are some examples:

• Research on animals: Researchers have found that fasting improves spatial memory (remembering where things are) and memory ability on a number of different tasks.

• Early research on humans shows that fasting might help older adults remember things better and might also help people with mild cognitive impairment.

Just a quick reminder: More long-term tests with people are needed to fully understand how bad these effects could be and how long they last.

The Motivation Corner

Even if you never want to try a multi-day fast, those shorter fasts that you do every day are great for your memory. Every time you say no to that late-night snack, think of it as an investment in your aging brain.

Easy Ways to Get the Most Out of the Benefits

• Make the most of those eating windows by focusing on whole, unprocessed foods, lean protein, and colorful veggies to get the most brain-healthy nutrition.

• Stay hydrated. Staying hydrated during fasts helps you concentrate and think more clearly, which makes your mind work better.

• Activities that improve memory: For a great brain workout, combine fasting with activities that improve memory, such as learning a language, playing an instrument, or doing puzzles.

While science is interesting, the magic really comes to life when you do things in real life. We will skip the scientific terms in this part and instead hear from real people who have experienced how fasting can improve their memory and overall brain power.

Stories from real people whose memories got better

People like you who have used fasting to improve their brain power can sometimes be the most inspiring proof. Even though everyone's experience is different, these stories show how fasting might improve remembering and thinking in surprising ways:

Story #1: Sarah, the Student Who Got Lost

'Head in the clouds' type that I've always been. It was normal for me to forget meetings, lose things, and have trouble remembering things for tests. I was trying to lose weight when I found out about intermittent fasting. What surprised me most was that my goal changed! All of a sudden, learning didn't seem so hard. Those annoying details stuck in my mind better, and I no longer had the crazy brain fog I had before tests.

Takeaway: Even short fasts can help you focus and make it easier to take in and remember what you've learned.

Story #2:

When I was in my early 60s, I realized that asking myself "where did I put my keys?" was becoming a daily bother. It made me a little worried about what could happen next. I wasn't sure if I should try intermittent fasting, but my daughter told me to. I thought it couldn't hurt. After a few months, the change is still slight but clear. I can remember more details about conversations, names of people more easily, and my mind usually works faster."

Possible Takeaway: Fasting might not get rid of all the memory problems that come with getting older, but it might slow down the process and help your brain feel fresh.

Story #3: Aisha, the Busy Business Owner

"Having my own business is great, but it's hard on the mind." It always felt like I had a million things open in my mind at once. Having longer fasts (24 to 36 hours) once or twice a week has surprised me with how calm and clear I feel. It's easier to sort through complicated data, remember important details without having to work too hard, and get through those days when you feel like your brain is too tired to do anything.

What You Might Learn: "Decision fatigue" might be helped by fasting, which could make it easier to think carefully and process information, even when you're under a lot of stress.

Important: These are just the author's own experiences; your own may be different. But they show that fasting can have effects on the brain that go beyond just remembering facts.

Different Ways, Same Results

See how each person found a way to fast that worked for them? Don't forget that it's all about customization! How do these stories relate to what we've already talked about?

• Sarah: She probably felt better when she limited her eating every day, even though she wasn't trying to go on longer fasts.

• Mark: His results show that extreme fasting might help with cognitive changes that come with getting older, but remember that consistency is key for the long term.

• Aisha: Shows how doing short fasts every so often can help people with busy lives think more clearly.

Is this really you?

Picture yourself a few months from now:

• Remembering meetings when your phone doesn't keep going off to remind you.

• Having the mental strength to do the things you've been putting off.

• Being sure of yourself and smart when you talk to people.

The Motivation Corner

It's simple to think that forgetfulness is just a part of "getting older." But these stories tell us that our brains can adapt and change in amazing ways, and fasting might be a way to help them do that!

Not to be Careless

Although inspiring, it's important to keep goals in check. Fasting is not a magic bullet that will erase all memory problems right away. It's like a puzzle piece that goes with other brain-healthy habits like eating well, exercising, and getting enough sleep.

Are you ready to find out what's possible?

Start with an easy 12-hour fast overnight or choose to eat only at certain times. Write down your thoughts in a "memory journal." Write down any changes that are good, even if they are small. Those wins will fuel your desire to keep learning what this amazing tool can do.

Memory-Boosting Exercises to Do While Fasting

Some types of exercise can help you change the way your brain works by making new connections and improving memory pathways. Fasting is like a spring cleaning for your brain. You can work out your body and your brain here:

The best thing for your brain is to work out.

Like fasting, exercise releases BDNF, which is a brain-boosting hero! In addition, it has these great benefits for memory:

• Makes the hippocampus bigger: Research has shown that regular exercise can make the hippocampus, the brain area that stores memories, bigger. It is thought that a bigger hippocampus means better remembering.

• Sparkly New Neurons: Exercise helps neurogenesis, which is the birth of new brain cells, especially in areas of the brain that are involved with remembering.

• Better Blood Flow: Working out makes your blood flow faster, which means more oxygen and nutrients get to your brain, which is exactly what it needs to remember things clearly.

When it comes to memory, not all exercise is the same. Any kind of action is great, but these seem especially good for your memory:

• To do aerobic exercise, you should take quick walks, jog, dance, or do anything else that makes your heart beat faster and makes you feel a little out of breath. Studies show that this type is very important for improving those brain areas.

• Exercises that build skills: When you learn new physical skills, like juggling, dancing, or even yoga, your brain has to work harder to make new links. Plus, it's enjoyable!

• Mindfulness Movement: Focused movement and breathwork, like tai chi, have been shown to lower stress and help older people remember things better.

The Routine with Extra Power: Memory Boosting Sets

Are you ready for some power pairs? Here's how to get the most brain-boosting benefits from these workouts and fasting:

Combination #1: The Memory Maker for the Morning

• Out of breath: Before your first meal, go for a 30- to 40-minute walk or do your best aerobic activity. Your brain will be ready to learn and focus with that BDNF boost and more blood flow.

• Fueling Up After a Workout: After a long fast, eat a healthy meal with protein and healthy fats to give your body and brain power.

Combination #2: A break for your mind

• The mid-fast focus is: When your energy level is stable after a longer fast, try learning a new skill for 20 to 30 minutes. This could be a dance routine, a tough yoga sequence, or even online brain games.

• Option for Mindful Movement: If you feel like focusing too much is draining, try focused gentle movement like tai chi or qigong, especially when you are calm and fasted.

Combination #3: Brain Boost Before Bed

• Wind-Down in the evening: Lessen your computer time an hour or two before bed by going for a walk and taking deep belly breaths. This calms the nervous system and gets the brain ready for a good night's sleep, which is important for remembering things.

The Motivation Corner

Don't see this as another thing you need to do. Think of it as a fun way to get even more out of fasting and treat your brain extra well. Here are some ways to keep yourself going:

• Begin little: Mindful moving for even 10 minutes is good for you! Work on making a habit that you stick to.

• Have fun: Try out a bunch of different workouts until you find one you like. That's what will help you keep going!

Combination #4 Team Up

Having a workout friend holds you accountable and makes the whole thing more fun.

Pay attention to your body and keep track of your progress. Just like when you fast, pay attention to how your body reacts to different kinds and intensities of exercise. Remember that this isn't about beating yourself up at the gym. It's about finding ways to move that make you happy and are good for your brain at the same time.

Remember to keep that journal ready! Pay attention to how these new exercise routines affect your ability to think clearly, sleep well, and learn new things. Your own views are strong motivators!

Chapter 7: Focus for the Win

Fighting Brain Fog and Improving Focus by Fasting

That annoying state of mind where your thoughts move slowly, your concentration is short, and getting anything done feels like slogging through mental mud. Brain fog can be caused by getting older, being stressed, or just feeling too busy. It can make it hard to do even the simplest things. It looks like fasting might help clear the fog.

How fasting can help clear your mind

Learn about the ways that fasting can clear your mind and help you concentrate:

• Energy Shift: Your body puts processing first when you're always eating. When you fast, your gut system gets a break. This frees up energy that can be used for other things, like thinking more clearly.

• Ketone Clarity: When you don't eat for a while, your body starts burning fat for energy, which makes ketones. Some people say that ketones make them feel more mentally focused and awake.

• Autophagy in Action: Remember how cells clean up after themselves? It turns out that it also helps get rid of brain junk! Getting rid of broken proteins and cell debris can help the brain work better and clear up foggy thinking.

• Less inflammation: Long-term inflammation is like having static electricity in your brain, making it hard to concentrate. It has been shown that fasting can reduce inflammation all over the body, even in the brain.

• Blood Sugar Balance: Brain fog can happen when your blood sugar goes up and down a lot. When you fast, your body naturally becomes more sensitive to insulin. This makes your blood sugar levels more stable and gives you more mental energy.

Things that cause brain fog: fasting can help

Let's look at some well-known causes of brain fog and how fasting can help:

• Too Much Stress: If you're constantly worried, your body makes a lot of cortisol, a stress hormone that makes it hard to think straight. Fasting, especially when done with tasks that lower stress, helps keep cortisol levels in check, which makes it easier to concentrate.

• Not getting enough sleep: Not getting enough sleep is bad for your brain! Fasting can help you sleep better, so when you wake up, your mind will be clear and ready to work.

• overload and Decision Fatigue: For many people, fasting makes them feel calm and clear, which can help them set priorities and fight the mental overload that causes brain fog.

What Could This Mean for You in the Real World?

Think of...

• Working on that hard project at work without getting stuck.

• Getting things done without getting tired in the middle of the day.
• Taking part in talks instead of just listening without contributing.

How to Get the Most Out of Focus-Boosting Activities

Here's how to get the most out of your fasts for concentration:

• Make the most of your fasting plan: Find the rhythm of fasting that gives you energy and clears your mind. For some, shorter fasts may work best, while for others, longer ones every once in a while are best.

• Eat well to learn well: Break your fast with protein, healthy fats, and colorful veggies, which are all whole foods that are good for your brain.

• Stay hydrated: being thirsty makes it very hard to concentrate! While you're fasting, drink water, and if you're fasting for a long time, you might want to add nutrients.

• Get even more benefits: do something that helps you concentrate while you're fasting, like a short meditation session, a quick walk in the park, or working on a creative project.

The Motivation Corner

Don't forget that even short, regular fasts can help you get out of brain fog! Each fast should be seen as a mental reset that gets rid of the noise and lets your real focus shine through.

Getting rid of a common myth

Some people are afraid that fasting will make them weak, dizzy, and unable to concentrate. This could happen at first as your body gets used to the changes, but for most people, it's followed by a rush of mental clarity and energy as their body gets better at using the energy it has saved.

An Important Note About Brain Fog

Even though fasting can be helpful, it's important to make sure that you don't have any underlying health problems that are making your brain fog last for a long time. If it's really bothering you, talk to your doctor about what might be causing it, like not getting enough nutrients, having a thyroid problem, or the side effects of your medications.

Are you ready to get rid of the fog?

Start fasting if you want to get rid of brain fog and replace it with laser-sharp focus. Keep track of your progress by writing down those times when you feel very clear or can focus for longer amounts of time. Don't forget to celebrate your wins; they will keep you motivated to fast regularly for a brain boost.

How to Stay Focused During and Between Fasts

These useful tips will help you focus on your goals while fasting and during your eating windows, so you can have a mentally productive day every day, no matter how long you've been fasting or how new you are to it.

While you're fasting: Get smart about your game. • Take on the challenge: Change how you think about hunger pangs from annoying distractions to signs that your body is switching food sources efficiently. This thought switch also helps you concentrate.

• Get your arsenal of distractions ready: Find things to do that will keep you from getting hungry or tired, like light exercise, a creative project, an audiobook, or important errands. Try different things to see what works best for you.

• Use the Power of Hydration: Clear thought is helped by drinking enough water. Having herbal drinks or water with a pinch of salt can also help you control your electrolytes and hunger.

• Change Your Scenery: If you find yourself getting mentally drowsy, going to a different room or taking a short walk outside can help you get back on track.

Mindful Moments: Take short breaks during your fast to be more aware of your thoughts and feelings. Pay attention to any physical signs of hunger, but don't think about them too much. Pay attention to your breath or do a quick check of your body. It helps you build "attention muscle."

In between fasts: Get your brain ready.

• Nourish with Purpose: Breaking fast with whole, organic foods gives you long-lasting energy and nutrients that help your brain. Put protein, healthy fats, and those very important fresh greens at the top of your list.

• Give up the sugar rush: Blood sugar spikes and crashes make it hard to concentrate. If you break your fast with sugary or highly processed carbs, your brain will be slow later on.

• Smart snacking (if you need to): To avoid brain fog in the middle of the day without slowing down your metabolism, try nuts, hard-boiled eggs, or plain yogurt with berries.

• Breaks That Help You Focus: If you want to improve your focus during breaks, don't mindlessly scroll through social media. Instead, do games, learn a new skill, or use brain-training apps.

Stacking Habits to Improve Focus

For a bigger effect, combine fasting with other good habits:
• Get up and move: You can focus and feel more energized with short bursts of exercise during or after a fast. A 10-minute walk or a few yoga moves can help.

• Meditate to Improve Your Mental Agility: Mindfulness practices make it easier to avoid distractions and stay focused, even when things get tough.

• The Nature Boost: Being outside calms the mind and helps you focus. Take a break from work and go for a walk in the park, or plan a walk in the park after a fast.

• Don't work too hard at night: For attention, you have to get regular, good sleep. Even though fasting can help you sleep better, good sleep hygiene is even better.

The Motivation Corner

You need time to build up your "focus muscles." Wait your turn and enjoy the trip! With each fast, you teach your body and mind to work together, which improves your ability to focus not only during fasts but also all day long.

It's important to personalize

Try different things to see what helps you focus the most. Here's how to unlock your ideal "Focus Formula:"

• The Best Time to Fast: If you have to choose, do you do best on 16:8 or 20-hour fasts? Find the beat that makes you feel good and keeps your mind sharp.

• Exercises in the morning vs. exercises in the evening: Is working out in the morning better for you after a fast, or is working out in the evening better? Schedule your workouts for times when they will help you get more done.

• Your Zen Zone: Where does the peace of mind feel the best? A quiet spot at home, a park bench, or a busy coffee shop? Pick out places where you can focus deeply.

Track your wins and make your strategy work better.

Write in a focus book! Note: • The times of day you can focus best; • Activities that help you avoid getting distracted while fasting;

• How window meals affect your ability to focus after a fast Being aware of yourself lets you improve your method! You could think of it as making your own "focus algorithm."

How to Play the Long Game: Being focused is a skill

You can get a lot out of fasting, but consistency is what will make the effects last. Accept that you are trying out new methods, that you are building your focus, and that you are enjoying the wins along the way. Having a sharp, clear mind is well worth the effort.

How to Stay on Task in Real Life

The world we live in is made to make us lose focus. With so many notifications and to-do lists, it's no wonder that staying on task feels like a fight all the time. But if you take the right steps, you can get back in charge of your workday (and life in general!) and stay focused the whole time.

TIP #1: The place where you live is very important.

Make your area as focused as possible:

• Get rid of the chaos: a place that looks jumbled makes you think jumbled. Get rid of everything on your desk except the things you need to do the job.

• Getting rid of noise: If you can, work in a quiet place. Headphones that block out noise or background music that helps you concentrate (like silent tracks or nature sounds) can make all the difference.

• Lighting Is Important: LED lights that are too bright can hurt your eyes and mind. Whenever you can, use natural light or buy a good work lamp that looks like sunlight.

Tip #2: Learn to control your digital pets.

To be honest, our devices are often the things that keep us from focusing. Use these strategies to take charge:

• Phone Out of Sight: Put your phone on quiet, turn off alerts that aren't necessary, and hide it in a drawer or bag. It's possible for your phone to unconsciously take your attention away just by being there.

• Website Blockers: If news or social media sites are distracting you, use apps that block websites during times when you need to concentrate.

Freedom and StayFocused are both great choices.

Planned Airplane Mode: If you need your phone close but can't stay away from the notifications, put it in airplane mode for a short time.

Tip #3: Control the To-Do Monster

To-do lists that are too long can stop you in your tracks. To break them down, do this:

• Brain Dump: Write down (or tap into your phone) all the things you need to do. This alone helps with mental overload.

• Three is a Power: Pick just three "must-do" things that you have to get done today. This helps you concentrate instead of feeling confused.

• Setting aside time: Schedule specific timeslots with brief breaks in between to refuel your focus.

Tip #4: Use the Power of Rituals

Do these things before you focus to let your brain know it's time to "go":

• The Dream Brew: Your pre-task beverage cue could be a certain type of tea, coffee, or energizing infused water.

• Soundtrack of Choice: Make a mix of music that helps you concentrate that you always play when you need to get things done.

• Quick Prep for the Body: You can get your energy back up to speed with a few minutes of deep breathing, stretching, or jumping jacks.

Micro-focus sessions are a great way to train your attention. Like building muscle, short bursts of attention can help you get better:

• The Pomodoro Method: Focus on your work for 25 minutes straight, then take a 5-minute break. Do this over and over. You can use a Pomodoro timer app to keep track of this method.

• Begin little: Focusing for even just 10 minutes straight is a win. As your mental strength grows, slowly add more time.

• One task at a time is king: That's not how our brains are wired to work. One thing at a time will help you get more done and keep your mind from getting tired.

The Motivation Corner

Staying on task is something you have to work at! Don't let occasional failures get you down. For the same reason you fast, think of it as a journey of constant self-improvement and discovery.

Celebrate every win, no matter how big or small.

• Did you finish a tough job without getting sidetracked? Good luck!
• Refused to look at your phone for an hour? That's a big step forward.
• Learned a difficult new skill by practicing it hard? You're really good at focusing!

The Effects of Focused Action on Other Things

Imagine all the great things you could do if you could focus as much as you could. Imagine how good it will feel to cross off big goals, easily pick up new skills, and finally get to the projects you've been putting off. Focus training pays off in ways that don't just happen at work.

Chapter 8: Stress Less, Smile More

What fasting does to your mood and anxiety

There's a state called "hangry" that happens when you're hungry and irritable at the same time. And here's the shocking part: fasting can have the opposite effect if you do it the right way. It can make you feel calmer, less anxious, and maybe even happier.

How fasting can change your mood

Let's look at the science behind this interesting link:

• Neurotransmitter Boost: When you fast, neurotransmitters (the chemicals that send messages in your brain) like serotonin and dopamine are changed. These chemicals are connected to mood regulation, drive, and reward feelings.

• BDNF Strikes Again: Remember that powerful protein we keep talking about? It does more than just improve memory; it also affects mood and can help people with anxiety and sadness feel better. It makes more of itself when you fast.

• Calming Ketones: Ketones are made when your body switches from using carbs for fuel to burning fat during a fast. Some people say that having high ketones makes them feel more focused and calm.

• Inflammation Tamer: Long-term inflammation makes it hard to relax and can make worry worse. Studies show that fasting may help lower inflammation in the brain and body as a whole.

• Builds resilience: Getting through those fasting hurdles can make you feel better about your own mental and physical strength. Feeling like you have control over your life in general makes it easier to deal with stress and worry.

Going from labs to real life: Possible Benefits

Even though we still don't know a lot about the long-term effects, this is what science says:

• Getting rid of anxiety: Early study suggests that fasting may help ease anxiety symptoms and make you feel calm.

• Mood booster: While it's not a sure thing, some studies show that regular fasting may improve your mood and make you less irritable.

• Better ability to handle stress: fasting might make you stronger against stress, lowering the overwhelming feelings that can cause worry and unhealthy cravings.

Important Things to Think About

It's not a magic bullet for mental health problems to fast. To understand, read this:

• Different people have different experiences; everyone reacts in their own way. If you already have a mental health problem, you should always talk to your doctor about fasting.

• Not a Stand-In Treatment: Think of fasting as ONE way to improve your mental health. It works best when combined with other healthy habits and, if necessary, professional help.

• Pay attention to your body: Fasting is not right for you if it makes your nervousness worse or causes you to eat in a disorderly way. You can improve your mental health in many other ways.

Motivation Corner: It's About Being Strong!

If your mood or anxiety goes up and down a lot, the idea that something as easy as planning when you eat could help is very empowering. Don't forget that fasting shows you that you are in charge—you can handle hunger and come out stronger. This alone can change the way you think in a big way.

How to Get the Most Out of Mood Enhancers

Are you ready to try it? Here's how to get the most out of your diet for mental health:

• Start Slowly and Stay Hydrated: If you want to avoid getting angry or anxious, especially at first, ease into fasting and make staying hydrated a top priority.

• Mindful Eating Windows: When you break a fast, eat whole foods that are good for you and give your brain the nutrients it needs to keep your mood stable.

• Do activities that calm you down at the same time. For an extra mood boost during fasts, try meditation, light exercise, or spending time in nature.

• Write down your mood: Keeping a mood record along with your fasting log can help you see patterns and benefits for yourself.

Why a holistic approach is important

Fasting may be one part of your health plan, but it works best when you add these other important parts as well:

• Enough Sleep: Not getting enough sleep is terrible for your mood. Fasting and getting better sleep together are very effective.

• Balanced nutrition: the foods you eat every day are a big part of controlling your mood. Going on a fast doesn't mean you can eat a lot of junk food.

Support System: Having a good support system will help you on your journey, whether it's professional help, a helpful friend, or online communities.

Are you ready to turn down the stress and find peace within yourself? This part talks about how fasting can change the way your body reacts to stress, making you feel calmer, stronger, and better prepared to deal with the unexpected things that happen in life.

Taking care of stress hormones and boosting calm

Stress is like your body's alarm system, which is there to help you stay alive when there are dangers around. In today's busy world, though, that alarm often gets stuck on high alert, filling your body with stress hormones that throw off your mental and physical health. What's good? You might need to fast to reset that alarm inside your head and find your calm center.

Tips for Getting Rid of Stress

Here are some ways that fasting can change the way you deal with stress:

• Controlling cortisol: Caffeine, which is your main stress hormone, naturally rises in the morning and falls throughout the day. This trend can be regulated by fasting, which may lower chronically high cortisol levels that cause anxiety and burnout.

• Neuroplasticity at Work: You can make your body more flexible by putting it under short-term stress (in a controlled way with fasting). In the long run, this makes you less likely to be stressed out, so you can handle problems as they come up instead of feeling overwhelmed all the time.

• Boosts your metabolism: Fasting can make it easier for your body to run on fat instead of carbs. Being able to change your metabolism can help you handle stress better, which can help you stay calm when things get crazy.

• Mind Over Matter: Being able to control your hunger pangs during a fast boosts your confidence, which in turn gives you more mental control and fewer urges to use unhealthy ways to deal with stress.

Benefits in the real world: Happier and less stressed

Fasting won't suddenly get rid of all your stress. But this is what it might give you:

• Inner Calm: That feeling of constant stress or being on edge slowly goes away and is replaced by a calm sense of well-being.

• Emotional Resilience: You don't get upset over small failures; instead, you get over them faster and with a stronger sense of "I can handle this."

• Less Reactivity: When problems come up, you think about how to handle them more carefully instead of responding quickly with anger or frustration.

For some reason, fasting might make you feel sleepy. More studies with real people are needed, but what has been learned so far points to an interesting possible effect:

• Stabilized Mood: Some studies show that fasting can help control mood swings and make people less irritable, which is a frequent sign of stress.

• Better Sleep: Getting enough sleep is a key part of dealing with stress. Fasting leads to deeper sleep, which causes a positive feedback loop.

• Lowers inflammation: Having too much cortisol can make inflammation worse, which can make health problems like worry worse as well. This inflammation might go down if you fast, which could help you handle stress better.

Tips for Getting the Most Out of Calm: Use these tips to get the most out of fasting's ability to relieve stress:

• Combo Power: Do something relaxing like yoga, meditation, or spending time in nature while fasting.

• Mindful Moments: Plan short awareness breaks into your fast to help you feel more grounded and calm.

• Put rest first: When you're on a long fast, don't try to keep up your normal energy output. Do more things that make you feel relaxed to help your body fight stress.

• Slowly break the fast: When you break your fast, eat light, healthy foods to keep your blood sugar from going up and down, which can make worry worse.

The Motivation Corner

It takes time to get your body used to worry! For the first few fasts, don't worry if you don't feel like a Zen master. Celebrate any small steps you take to feel calmer and stronger. If you keep at it, those small steps will add up to big changes.

Why being self-aware is important

Pay attention to your body! This is where careful observation is very important:

• Does fasting calm or rouse you? For some, fasting helps them concentrate and feel calm. For some, especially those who are new to fasting, it can make them feel more irritable for a short time.

• Find a place to relax: You might feel best after a short fast, or you might feel calmer after a longer fast. You are the only one who can find what works!

• Stress Made Worse? Definitely stop fasting if it makes your stress levels much higher or your nervousness worse. Respect what you've been through and look into kinder ways to deal with stress instead.

A Strong Helper, Not a Magic Cure

Remember that fasting is one way to deal with stress. It works best when joined with these important habits:

• Doing regular exercise: Moving your body is a great way to relieve stress. Find a way to move that you enjoy and do it every day.

A good night's sleep: It's important to get enough sleep so that your body and mind can fully recharge. This will help you deal with worry better.

• Ask for help: If you're dealing with long-term worry or stress, you should get help from a professional, like a therapist or your doctor.

There is a strong link between your mental health and the general health of your brain. This is a very important idea that is often overlooked. Get rid of the idea that they are two different things! Knowing this link gives you the power to make decisions that are good for both your happiness and your brain's long-term health.

Why mental health is important for brain health in general

Your brain is in charge of more than just your memories and thoughts. It also controls your emotions, your stress response, and all the other complex processes that keep you alive. It makes sense that if your mental health gets worse, your brain health can get worse too (and the other way around!).

Problems with mental health can hurt the brain in bad ways Here are some ways that long-term mental health problems can hurt your brain:

• Changes in the brain's structure: Less brain volume in parts of the brain that are important for memory and controlling emotions is linked to mental illnesses like sadness and anxiety.

• More swelling and pain: Mood disorders and long-term worry can make inflammation worse all over the body, including in the brain. This inflammation hurts brain cells and makes it harder to think clearly.

• Risk of Alzheimer's and Dementia: Studies show that untreated sadness and long-term anxiety raise the chance of getting Alzheimer's and dementia later in life.

Brain chemicals, like serotonin and dopamine, can become out of balance, which can lead to mood disorders. Mood disorders can affect a lot of things, from drive to sleep.

The Vicious Cycle: How the Mind Affects the Brain

You can go either way! In the same way that mental health problems affect the brain, changes in the health of your brain can also make you more likely to have mental health problems:

• Head injuries: Even mild concussions can change your mood for a long time and make you more likely to develop sadness and anxiety.

• Not getting enough nutrients: To work at its best, your brain needs certain minerals and vitamins. Deficiencies can make you feel down, tired, and cause brain fog.

• Changes that come with getting older: As you get older, your brain naturally changes in ways that can make you more likely to have mood swings, be irritable, and feel like you're losing your mind.

• Long-Term Illnesses: Diabetes and heart disease both lower the amount of blood that gets to the brain. This makes it more likely that you will have mental health problems or lose your memory.

It's important to remember that this doesn't mean that every bad day means you have major brain damage or that you can stop mental health problems from happening. There's more to it than that! But it's clear that knowing this link has power.

Good news: your brain can handle a lot!

Don't let this scare you; it's meant to get you excited! Your brain can fix itself in amazing ways, and taking care of your mental health is one of the best things you can do to keep your brain working well for years to come.

Putting the Power of Prevention to Use

This is where things get interesting: the same good habits that make you feel better also protect your brain:

• Fasting for the Win: Fasting may help protect your brain from damage, which could lower your risk of neurodegenerative diseases over time. It may also help with worry and mood stability.

• Less stress means less brain stress: long-term stress hurts brain cells. Putting relaxation skills, mindfulness, and healthy ways to deal with stress at the top of your list is a gift to both your present and future selves.

• Give your brain food: A diet full of fruits, veggies, and healthy fats gives your brain and mood the building blocks they need to work at their best.

• Movement is Magic: Exercise increases blood flow, helps new neurons grow, and improves mood—it's like a magic bullet for the brain.

Connection with other people: Strong ties lower stress, increase chemicals in the brain that make you feel good, and may even lower the risk of cognitive decline.

The Motivation Corner

It is simple to think of "brain health" as something you only have to worry about as you get older. But the truth is that every healthy choice you make today, every time you take charge of your stress, and every time you put your mood first, you're building a mind that will be smarter, happy, and stronger for decades to come. That's the best way to love yourself!

When You Should Get Help from a Pro

Self-care is important, but it's NOT a replacement for professional help if you're having a hard time:

• Don't wait until things go wrong: It's not a sign of weakness to get help for things like sadness, anxiety, or other problems. It's better to get help right away.

• Therapy trains the brain: Therapy trains people how to deal with stress, change harmful ways of thinking, and become emotionally strong. It's like working out your brain!

• Your doctor is on your side: Talk freely with your doctor about your mental health. They can look for deeper causes and give you a range of personalized treatment choices.

Chapter 9: Guarding Against Decline

Fasting for Reducing the Risk of Alzheimer's and Other Dementias

It's normal to feel scared about losing our memories and our freedom as we age. In spite of this, new research gives us hope: fasting, when done in a planned way, may lower your risk of getting these terrible diseases. Understanding this research gives you the power to make choices that will improve your brain health in the long term, but it's not a surefire way to avoid getting dementia.

How fasting can help you keep your precious memories safe Let's look at the different ways that taking breaks to eat might help protect your brain against decline:

• Autophagy: Remember our favorite cleaner-up team for cells? It works even better when you fast, getting rid of misfolded proteins that can lead to diseases like Alzheimer's. It's like getting rid of the trash in your head!

• Less inflammation: Long-term inflammation is a cause of many diseases that come with getting older, including brain health decline. By lowering inflammation, fasting can protect those brain cells.

• Ketone Power: Your body makes ketones when you're fasting. In some ways, these might help your neurons, which could slow down the damage caused by Alzheimer's.

• Boosting Brain Powerhouses: Fasting makes the body make more BDNF, which helps new brain cells grow. This makes the structure of your brain stronger, which makes it more durable.

• Metabolic Reset: Fasting makes insulin work better, which lowers your risk of diabetes, which is a big risk factor for Alzheimer's and cognitive decline.

What we know so far: Potentially good but cautious

This is the most interesting study on fasting and preventing Alzheimer's that has been done on animals. It looks very good, but here's what we need to keep in mind:

• Mice Aren't People: Studies on animals help us understand the effects, but we need more long-term studies on people right away.

• There Isn't Just One Size That Fits All: How long should you fast for, and what kind is best for brain health? Every person may get a different answer.

• Lifestyle Is Most Important: Fasting is a strong tool, but it won't fix a bad way of life in general. It's most effective when used with other safety steps.

Lessons for Real Life: Reasons to be hopeful

While we wait for more clear studies on humans, the science we already have gives you strong reasons to think about fasting as part of your routine:

• Potential for early intervention: If fasting works, it could change everything, especially for people who have a family history of memory loss.

• The Power to Stop: If fasting only slightly lowers your risk, that's still a big deal when it comes to a disease like Alzheimer's.

• Brain Boost All Around: Fasting has many benefits besides preventing dementia. You're fighting inflammation, making your brain stronger, and improving the health of your metabolism. All of these are great things!

The Motivation Corner

Diseases like Alzheimer's can make you feel like you have no control over them. The cool thing about fasting is that it puts YOU back in charge of your health in the long run. It's not just about science; it's also about giving people power.

Using fasting along with other safety measures

When you fast along with these habits that are good for your brain, it works even better:

• The MIND Diet: This plan focuses on eating lots of fresh greens, berries, nuts, and fatty fish, which have all been linked to better brain health as you age.

• Plan your workouts: both cardio and muscle training are good for your brain. For long-lasting effects, do things you enjoy.

• Exercise your mind: learn a new language, play word games, or pick up a hard sport to keep your neurons firing.

• Sleep Sanctuary: Make deep, healing sleep a priority. This is when your brain cleans up in important ways that may lower your risk of Alzheimer's.

• Things that relieve stress: Stress that you can't control is bad for your brain. Find good ways to deal with things that are bothering you.

Important Don't Forget

Talk to your doctor about fasting if you have a family history of Alzheimer's or dementia. They can give you specific advice on how to safely and successfully use it as part of a larger plan to stay healthy.

Protecting brain cells and boosting longevity

It's not just about the number of years we want to live. It's about being able to enjoy the most important things in life while still being at full strength. This is where it gets really exciting to understand the link between fasting and living a long life.

How fasting might make you live longer and be healthier Here are some ways that fasting might help you not only live longer, but also live BETTER for longer:

• Cellular Rejuvenation: Autophagy does more than just clean out your brain. It takes care of your whole body, getting rid of old, broken cells and making room for new ones. On a cellular level, this renewal slows down some signs of age.

• Telomere Power: Think of telomeres as caps that protect your genes. As they age, they naturally get shorter. According to some research, fasting might slow down this process, which would keep your cells "young" for longer.

• Turning on genes linked to longevity: Studies show that fasting might turn on genes linked to longevity, which would speed up your body's natural repair processes.

• Better metabolic health: Fasting lowers the chances of getting age-related diseases like diabetes, heart disease, and some cancers, so you not only live longer but also better.

• Fights inflammation: Long-term inflammation supports a lot of the decline that comes with getting older. It helps keep it in check, which is good for your body and brain.

Studies on animals vs. potential for people

A lot of the ground-breaking study has been done on animals, where scientists have seen that fasting routines can significantly extend life spans. Keeping realistic goals in mind, here's why that's inspiring:

• Proof of Concept: Studies on animals show us how the biological processes might work. Now we need to catch up with the studies on people.

•It's Not Just About Very Long Length: Even if fasting doesn't add decades to your life, the goal of increasing your health span—those years of being joyful and free—is a strong and inspiring one.

• Translation in Progress: Scientists are working hard to turn what they've learned from studying animals into safe, long-term ways for people to fast that will help them live longer.

Corner for Motivation: Quality, Not Just Amount, Is Important

No one wants to spend a long time just existing. What makes fasting really powerful is that it can help you thrive in old age, with a sharp mind, a healthy body, and the energy to keep doing the things you enjoy.

You can start at any time.

The great thing about fasting is that you might feel better no matter when you start. This is how it breaks down:

• Early Birds, Big Wins: Starting to fast, even for short periods of time, when you are an adult sets your body up for healthy aging and may even help you live longer.

• Mid-Life Adopters: It's still not too late if you're middle-aged! Fasting can help reduce inflammation and improve the health of your metabolism.

• Seniors Save Money: Even if you start fasting later in life, it could help your cells renew themselves, protect your brain health, and raise markers of good aging, making your later years better.

Fasting is a way of life.

This "fountain of youth" really works in the long run. Don't think of fasting as a quick fix, but as a way to slow down the aging process. When used with these basics, it works best:

• The Longevity Diet: Focus on whole foods, lots of veggies, and lean protein. Think of it like the Mediterranean diet, but with fewer meals!

• Move as Medicine: Do things that make you feel good that you have to include them in every part of your life!

• Protect Your Sleep: You need deep sleep to heal your cells and stay healthy in general. Poor sleep speeds up the aging process.

• The worry Factor: Long-term worry shortens telomeres and makes you age faster than you should. Managing stress in a good way is very important.

• Connection to the community: Strong relationships are good for your physical and mental health at any age, so enjoy the extra years you have.

How to Understand the Most Recent Research

Large-scale studies on fasting to avoid disease in humans take time, but here are some exciting areas that scientists are looking into right now:

Focus Area #1: Diets that mimic fasting and brain health

• The Research: Studies are looking into how FMDs, which last for about 5 days, might affect memory loss, brain age, and the risk of getting Alzheimer's disease.

• What's exciting about it is that FMDs might make some of the benefits of fasting easier to get while reducing the need for long-term food restriction.

• What We're Waiting For: Long-term studies with humans are needed to find out if the positive benefits last and if certain FMD protocols are best for protecting the brain.

Focus Area #2: The Best Time to Start Intermittent Fasting

• The Research: Scientists are looking at different fasting routines (16:8 vs. alternate-day fasting, etc.) to see which ones will help fight aging and protect the brain the most.

• Why it's exciting: this makes fasting more flexible so that it can fit the needs of each person. Some people do better with longer fasts, while others get amazing results from shorter daily ones.

• What We're Waiting For: We need to find out if there's a "dose-response relationship"—does longer fasting times always mean more benefits, or does it get less useful after a while?

Focus Area #3: Fasting and Signs of Aging

• The Research: Scientists are looking at how fasting affects biomarkers such as telomere length, inflammation, and metabolic markers. This is helping them figure out how fasting protects cells.

• Why it's exciting: this is more than just better symptoms. It lets us see changes that happen with getting older at the cellular level, which could show how fasting slows down the aging process itself.

• What we're interested in: Studies that keep track of people for a long time to see if the changes in those biomarkers lead to lower rates of cognitive loss and diseases that come with getting older in the long run.

Area of Focus #4: Customized Fasting

• About the Study: Researchers are beginning to look into how genes and pre-existing health conditions affect how people react to fasting and what routines work best for them.

• What's exciting about this is that it opens the door to personalized fasting advice, since the same method won't work best for everyone, just like with medicine.

• What We're Waiting For: Studies with bigger, more varied groups of people and information on how personal factors may favor certain fasting styles (like eating less often vs. fasting for longer periods of time).

You are ahead of the curve, so use this as motivation.

You're already miles ahead just because you want to know how fasting can help you live longer. Don't forget that fasting safety puts you in the lead when it comes to proactive health, even if we don't have all the answers yet.

How to Stay Informed and Gain Power

Want to keep track of how this study is changing quickly? How to do it:

• Sources You Can Trust: You can find study summaries on trustworthy websites, such as those of the National Institutes of Aging (https://www.nia.nih.gov/) or well-known research universities.

• Stay away from hype: Watch out for websites that offer miracle cures or make science sound too easy. Look for expert insight that is fair and balanced.

• Community Power: Join online forums or groups where people talk about their fasting experiences and new studies in a responsible, fact-based way.

A Word About Patience and Putting Things in Perspective:

Science takes time, especially when it comes to hard topics like how to live longer and avoid getting sick. The main point is this:

• It's not a goal, but a journey: Don't give up if we don't have all the answers yet. Pay attention to the changes you CAN make to your lifestyle right now, knowing that they will help you be healthier in the future.

• Big steps forward are on the way: With more people interested in and funding for study in this area, it's clear that more ground-breaking discoveries are on the way!

Chapter 10: Autophagy: Your Brain's Cleanup Crew

Explaining Autophagy in Simple Terms

Think of your mind as a busy city. Every day, people get new knowledge, get rid of old memories, and do hard tasks. But trash builds up, just like in any busy city. That's where autophagy comes in. It's like having a cleaning crew in your brain that works nonstop to keep everything running nicely!

Autophagy: The Powerhouse of Cellular Recycling

It is pronounced "aw-TAH-fah-gee," which means "self-eating" in Greek. It might sound scary, but it's actually a very important cellular process that keeps your brain and body working well. How it works:

• Cellular Housekeeping: Over time, your cells collect broken proteins, organelles that don't work (like little factories inside your cells), and even waste from normal cellular processes. Autophagy finds this "junk" and packs it up to be thrown away.

• The Recycling Center: These packages are then sent to lysosomes, which are special parts inside cells. Lysosomes are like tiny recycle plants that take old, broken parts and break them down into their basic building blocks.

• Reuse and repurpose: Your cells then use these building blocks to make new, healthy parts. Like taking apart an old bike and putting together a new one from the parts!

Why autophagy is important for brain health

As we get older, autophagy normally works less well. This can cause a buildup of dead cells, which can make it harder to think clearly and can even cause brain inflammation and neurodegenerative illnesses like Alzheimer's. The good news, though? According to research, we might be able to protect our brains and keep them working at their best for longer by speeding up autophagy.

Fasting: The Booster for Autophagy

An interesting twist is that fasting, especially irregular fasting, seems to be a strong way to start autophagy. When your body doesn't get any food for a while, it speeds up the process of renewing cells. At its core, the body says, "Okay, since outside resources are limited, let's clean house and make good use of what we have!"

Why a clean cellular environment is good for you

By doing things like fasting that boost autophagy, you might be:

• Improving the health of brain cells: brain cells work better and more quickly when their environment is clean.

• Lessening inflammation: Autophagy gets rid of dead cells and other debris that can cause inflammation, which is a big cause of brain decline with age.

• Improving Cognitive Function: If you get rid of more "junk" from your system, your brain may be able to remember things better, concentrate better, and think more clearly overall.

Keep in mind that the study of autophagy and brain health is still very new and has a lot of potential. To fully understand the long-term effects, more studies with real people are needed.

Remember that it's never too late to start.

If autophagy hasn't been a top priority for your brain lately, the good news is that you can make it work better by making some changes to the way you live. You can fast, but it's not the only thing that can help you. Here are some more things you can do to help your brain's natural cleaning crew:

• Work out regularly: Cardiovascular exercise, in particular, helps your body's autophagy process all over, including in your brain.
• Good Sleep: While you sleep, your brain can work on cleaning up cells, which includes autophagy.

• Deal with stress: long-term stress throws off autophagy. Relaxation methods should be a top priority for maintaining a healthy cellular environment.

Why fasting helps the brain get rid of waste and recycle cells

If you think of fasting as a reset button, it means that your brain can clean itself out completely again. This amazing change takes place in a few steps, which are as follows:

Stage 1: Changing Gears: From Building to Cleaning

When you eat all the time, your body is busy with processes that help it grow. This is what your body tells you during a fast: "Okay, no new resources coming in. Time to save and reuse what we already have."

• Sense the Change: Your cells can tell when your food and energy levels change while you're fasting. This sets off a chain of messages that tell them to change gears.

• Not as much building, but more upkeep: When you slow down processes like growth and cell division, your cells can use their energy to clean up and fix things.

Stage 2: is called "Autophagy, Fully Ahead!"

Autophagy is activated when you fast, but it works even faster when you don't eat. How to do it:

• Putting together "Isolation Squads": Inside your cells, something called an autophagosome forms. It has two membranes and a special structure. Think of them as little cleanup teams that are checking out your brain cells.

• Trash Tagging: These autophagosomes find broken proteins, worn-out mitochondria (the powerhouses of your cells), and other junk that needs to be thrown away.

• Taking it to the "Recycling Center": The autophagosomes take in the trash and move it to the lysosomes, which are the recycling plants we talked about earlier.

Stage 3: Getting rid of waste and recovering resources

There are strong enzymes inside the lysosomes that break down the cell waste. This is where the real magic takes place:

- Breaking It Down: The waste is broken down into its basic parts, such as amino acids, fatty acids, DNA, and more.

• New Parts: Your cells use these recovered building blocks to make new proteins, fix broken structures, and even make brand-new mitochondria that are healthy. Talk about long-term use!

Why It's Important: The Benefits for Brain Health

Let's talk about how this cleaning of cells can help your brain in the real world:

Keeping your brain safe from "gunk": fasting may help autophagy work better, which may stop the buildup of misfolded proteins that are linked to Alzheimer's and Parkinson's.

• Controlling inflammation: Getting rid of damaged cell parts helps lower inflammation, which is a major cause of brain fog and cognitive loss.

• Neuron Power-Up: Autophagy helps new brain cells grow, memories form, and general cognitive function by giving cells recycled materials.

Focus on Research: Fasting and the Brain

A lot of the research is done on animals, but the findings are very encouraging:

• Studies with animals: Fasting increases autophagy in the brain, lowers inflammation in the brain that comes with getting older, boosts cognitive function, and may even slow the development of neurodegenerative diseases in mice.

• New Human Research: Early studies show that fasting might make you smarter and lower your risk of brain loss that comes with getting older.

Motivation Corner:

You're giving your inner recycling system more power. It's not just your body that goes without food when you fast; you also tell your brain cells to do important maintenance and repair work. Think of fasting as a way to get the most out of your body's natural anti-aging system.

Other Autophagy Allies Besides Fasting

Fasting is a strong speed booster, and these habits also help autophagy work at its best:

• Limit on calories: Even cutting back on calories in a mild way can boost autophagy, which is good for brain health and long life.

• "Autophagy-Boosting" Compounds: Resveratrol and green tea are two examples of naturally occurring compounds that may help repair and rebuild cells.

• Targeted Therapies: Researchers are looking into drugs that could specifically increase autophagy. This could lead to new ways to treat neurodegenerative diseases.

Are you ready to take the next step in recycling in your brain? Always do the same thing when it comes to autophagy. Having regular fasts, even if they are short, gives your brain's cleaning crew a regular workout that improves performance and helps your health in the long run. It will be good for you in the long run.

The Proof That Brains Work

"Spring Cleaning" is about autophagy, which is your brain's cleaning crew.
Remember that autophagy is like a small trash and recycling system in your brain. Here's more about the science behind how everything works:

The Important People: Come Meet the Molecules

A number of important chemicals control this complicated process. Think of them as the bosses of your cleaning crew:

• AMPK: Your cells' energy monitor. It turns on when the body is fasting or has low energy, telling it to save resources and start cleaning mode.

• mTOR: The one who controls growth. When there are lots of nutrients, mTOR helps cells grow. But when you're starving, it stops, letting autophagy take over.

• Transcription Factors: These proteins decide how genes are expressed. Certain transcription factors turn on genes that help make the autophagosomes, which are like clean-up crews.

Clean Up Step by Step: How It Performs

Let's look at those important steps of the autophagy spring cleaning session:

The first step is for AMPK to pick up on the change in energy levels during fasting and send the message, "Time to clean house!" At the same time, the growth manager, mTOR, gets a short break.

Autophagosome Formation: A phagophore, a double-membrane structure, starts to surround the trash that needs to be recycled. It's kind of like taking out the trash.

Expanding and Targeting: The phagophore gets bigger and takes in the "tagged" waste, making an autophagosome, a sealed bag of cell debris.

Off to Recycling: The autophagosome joins with a lysosome, which is your cell's recycling plant, and strong enzymes start breaking down the contents.

Rebuild and refuel: The basic building blocks, like amino acids, fatty acids, and so on, are sent back into the cell to be used for fixing cells, making energy, or building new structures. Why it's SO important to clean your brain

For better health, all of this spring cleaning comes down to one thing: cells that are clean and working well.

• Protecting Against Protein Gunk: Autophagy gets rid of misfolded or clumped proteins that are linked to Alzheimer's, Parkinson's, and Huntington's diseases.

• Healthy mitochondria = energized brain cells: Autophagy gets rid of old or broken mitochondria and makes room for new, healthy ones to grow. This keeps your brain cells active.

• Less inflammation: Getting rid of the dead cells and other waste reduces inflammation, which is a big reason why our brains get worse with age and cause brain fog.

Autophagy in Action: A Look at the Research

The study that shows autophagy is linked to brain health is very exciting:

• Preventing Neurodegeneration: Research shows that neurodegenerative diseases related to getting older are linked to impaired autophagy. Improving autophagy could be a treatment goal.

• Fasting to Focus: Even short-term fasting improves brain autophagy pathways and may help people and animals think more clearly and remember things.

• More Than the Brain: Autophagy isn't just for the brain! It's an important process all over your body, and it helps your metabolism, immune system, and general health.

That's right, you do have the power!

Mind cells are like little homes that need regular care. Autophagy works like those super-efficient cleaners who come in, clear, fix things up, and make everything work better. The cool thing is that you can speed up this process, which gives your brain the best chance to stay strong and sharp over time.

Why regular maintenance is important

It's not like you would spring clean your house once a year. Autophagy works best when you do it every day. Good news:

Fasting is a Star Player because it is a strong way to start autophagy, which gives your brain a deep cleaning boost.

Strategies for the long term: Along with calorie restriction and exercise, short, regular fasts keep those cleanup teams busy all the time.

Chapter 11: Boosting BDNF: Growing New Brain Cells

Why BDNF is important for brain health

This is a protein called Brain-Derived Neurotrophic Factor. It is found in your brain and nerve system. It's kind of like boosted brain fertilizer and is in charge of:

1. The growth and development of brain cells: The process of making new neurons (brain cells) is called neurogenesis, and BDNF helps it happen. Brain cells are always being made, even when we are adults. BDNF helps cells grow!

2. Making connections stronger: BDNF makes synapses stronger, which are the places where brain cells talk to each other. Stronger synapses help you think and remember things better and faster. They also help you learn more effectively.

3. Safety and Repair: BDNF protects your nerves from damage caused by stress, toxins, and normal wear and tear that comes with getting older. It's a defense mechanism built into your brain.

As to why you should be interested in your BDNF levels More BDNF is linked to a lot of great brain benefits, including

• Better memory: BDNF is especially important in the hippocampus, which is the memory center of your brain. It's possible that increasing BDNF could help you make, store, and recall memories.

• Mood booster: Anxiety and sadness are linked to low BDNF. Increasing it works like a natural sedative, helping to keep your mood in check and making you stronger emotionally.

• Defense Against Decline: Research shows that BDNF might help lower the chance of neurodegenerative diseases like Parkinson's and Alzheimer's.

• Better learning: BDNF makes brain cells more flexible, which is a process known as neuroplasticity. This helps you learn new things faster, remember them better, and get good at them more quickly.

What Changes Your BDNF Levels?

Some of you can change how much BDNF your brain makes, which is pretty cool. What helps, and what gets in the way, are these:

Boosters for BDNF:

Fasting: Yes, fasting does raise BDNF. This may be one of the main ways it helps your brain!

• Exercise: Regular exercise, especially cardio, boosts BDNF, which helps explain why staying busy is good for your brain.

• Healthy Fats: Omega-3-rich fatty fish and other foods like them are good for brain health, and upping BDNF may be one reason for this.

• Sunlight: Getting vitamin D from the sun might help your BDNF levels.

Busters for BDNF:

• Long-Term Stress: Because high amounts of cortisol block BDNF, long-term stress is terrible for your brain health.

• Inflammation: When the body is inflamed as a whole, BDNF levels drop in the brain.

• Not getting enough sleep: Not getting enough sleep lowers your BDNF, which could make you feel bad and cause brain fog.

BDNF creation goes down when you eat a lot of processed foods, sugar, and unhealthy fats.

Thought For The Day: You Can Boost Your Brain Power

You have a lot of power when you know you can change your BDNF levels! Every good choice you make is like putting money into a stronger, more resilient brain. You are building a better brain from the inside out.

BDNF and fasting: A Powerful Pair

Researchers have found that fasting can raise BDNF levels by a large amount. That's so cool for these reasons:

• Memory and Focus: The rise in BDNF may help explain why many people say they have better memory and focus while fasting or after.

• Anti-Aging Shield: Since fasting raises BDNF, it may give your brain an extra layer of defense against the cognitive loss that comes with getting older.

• A Long-Term Plan: Fasting may raise BDNF levels over time if done with other healthy habits, which will have long-lasting effects for the brain.

Getting the Best Results: Besides Fasting

Get the most out of that BDNF boost by using these techniques along with fasting:

• Mindful Movement: If you work out before, during, or after your fast, you might make even more BDNF.

• Brain-Boosting Foods: Omega-3s, leafy greens, and bright vegetables can help your body make more BDNF.

• Dealing with stress: Because worry lowers BDNF, make time for healthy ways to relax, like meditation or spending time in nature.

Are you ready to learn more?

How fasting increases, the production of BDNF

Do not forget that BDNF is like Miracle-Gro for your brain. It protects your brain cells from damage, makes new ones grow, and improves the ones you already have. Amazingly, fasting seems to work like a natural switch that makes your body better at making BDNF!

When you fast, your BDNF levels go up.

Let's look at the science behind how not eating leads to brain gains:

• Sensing Energy Shifts: When you fast, your cells notice that the amount of energy available changes. This sets off a chain of signals that tells your body to go into a mode that protects and repairs itself.

• BDNF Comes to the Rescue: Increasing the production of BDNF is a key part of this protective reaction. You can think of it as your brain getting stronger while there isn't enough food.

• Cellular "Remodeling": The BDNF boost helps neurogenesis (the growth of new neurons) and makes connections stronger between brain cells that are already there. It's just your brain getting used to things and working better!

• Benefits That Last: Studies show that the rise in BDNF that happens when you fast may last even after you start eating again, which could mean that you continuc to bcncfit your brain in thc long run.

Keep an eye on the evidence: what the research says

A lot of the research is done on animals, but the findings are very encouraging:

• Studies on Animals: Studies on animals regularly show that different fasting plans raise BDNF levels in the brain, especially in important parts like the hippocampus.

• Early Research on People: Early studies show that fasting may also raise BDNF levels in people, which could improve brain function and mood stability.

Why this is important: Brain Benefits in the Real World

Putting higher amounts of BDNF into real-life terms, this is what it could mean for you:

• Sharper Thinking: Higher levels of BDNF may be one reason why fasting makes people more focused, helps their minds work faster, and improves their general cognitive abilities.

• Better memory: Since BDNF is important for the hippocampus (your memory center), fasting may help with both short-term and long-term memory.

• Mood booster: A lack of BDNF has been linked to sadness in studies. The BDNF-boosting effect of fasting might help improve mood and mental strength.

• Long-Term defense: By increasing the production of BDNF, fasting may help protect against some of the cognitive loss that comes with getting older and may also help the brain stay healthy for longer.

Corner for Motivation: You're Making Your Brain Better!

When you make it through a fast, you do more than just burn calories. You are encouraging your brain to change and grow! That hunger pain has a whole new meaning now that you know this, doesn't it?

Running a fast isn't a magic bullet.

Remember that BDNF is only one piece of the brain health puzzle. Here's how to get the most out of them:

• Consistency Is Key: Regular fasting, even if it's just for a short time, helps keep your BDNF levels high.

• It takes a team: When you fast along with other habits that increase BDNF, like exercise, sleep, and a brain-healthy diet full of omega-3s and leafy veggies, the effects are stronger. • Take care of your stress: Long-term stress can undo all the good work that BDNF does. Managing your stress should be a top concern, especially if you're fasting.

What the BDNF Means

It's more than just a research interest that fasting and BDNF are linked. Reminding yourself that you have a surprising amount of control over your brain health is very powerful.

It's encouraging to know that you can actively make that brainpower character that protects and improves your brain function!

Neuroplasticity: Making sure your brain can change

Scientists used to think that brain growth peaked in childhood and then slowly slowed down as people got older. Everything changed, though, when neuroplasticity was discovered. It turns out that your brain is much more flexible than we thought. It can change its shape and function based on what you do, even as you get older.

Neuroplasticity: How Your Brain Changes and Grows

How it works:

• Wiring up the networks again: When you learn a new skill, go through a new experience, or break a bad habit, your brain makes new links between neurons and strengthens old ones. It's kind of like adding new roads and lanes for traffic in your brain.

• "Use It or Lose It" means that brain links you don't use often get cut off. This constant rebuilding makes your brain more efficient, so it can focus more on the things you do regularly.

• Neurons that Fire Together, Wire Together: When you practice a new skill or your brain cells fire in a coordinated manner over and over, the connections between them get stronger. This makes the networks work better.

Why neuroplasticity is really important!

The thought that your brain can change as you do changes what it means to learn new things throughout your life. Neuroplasticity changes everything because:

• No matter how old you are, your brain can still learn new things and build on what you already know. Don't think that you can't think of anything! It might take some more practice.

• Protection and Resilience: Neuroplasticity is the brain's way of changing to fit its surroundings, even when those surroundings are stressful. When things go wrong, a brain that is more flexible can handle them better.

• Recovery from a Stroke or Brain Injury: Neuroplasticity is what lets people get back the functions they lost after a stroke or brain injury. Their brains learn new ways to do those things and change themselves.

• Cognitive Longevity: Using your brain and encouraging neuroplasticity may help protect you from cognitive loss that comes with getting older and keep your mind sharp for longer.

Putting Neuroplasticity to Good Use

You don't have to just hope for the best, which is good news. If you take the right steps, you can actively improve your neuroplasticity!

• Get out of your comfort zone: Stop doing what you're doing! Take a dance class, learn a new language, play an instrument, or travel to places you've never been before. The point is to give your brain new experiences that help it grow.

• Pay attention: Focused practice of a skill improves the connections between brain cells more than doing other things at the same time. Keep the other things away while you learn!
• Workouts for your mind: puzzles, brain games, and memory drills are like focused resistance training for certain brain skills.

• Fasting to Focus: One reason why fasting might help improve neuroplasticity is that it makes it easier to concentrate and think clearly.

Corner for Motivation: Putting money into it is not a sprint! Improving your neuroplasticity won't make you smarter fast. The goal is to keep your mind constantly interested, open to new experiences, and flexible. You're building a brain that can handle anything life throws at it every time you leave your comfort zone or learn something new.

Neuroplasticity and BDNF: A Dynamic Pair

Do you remember that brain-boosting hero called BDNF? It is very important for learning!

• A base for growth: BDNF helps new neurons form and makes the connections between old cells stronger. You could think of it as making the conditions right for neuroplastic change to happen.

• Fasting Makes the Fire Burn: Since fasting raises BDNF, it may make your brain more flexible, so you can get more out of new experiences and difficult learning chances.

The Neuroplasticity Way of Life

To make neuroplasticity a part of your everyday life, do these things:

• Take on the challenge: Think of problems and failures as chances to learn and grow. Think of those hard times as exciting chances for your brain to grow.

• Enjoy the little wins: Did you remember the name of a new person? Learned how to do a tricky dance move? Celebrate your small wins; they will keep you going and show your brain that this flexibility thing is worth it.

• Give yourself time and kindness: When it comes to rewiring your brain, change doesn't happen fast. Getting a little angry is normal! Not just the end goal, but also the process of learning.

Are you ready to take on the task of learning new things all the time and making your brain very flexible? Don't forget that the trip itself is a great way to improve your brain, and it will work for ycars to comc!

Chapter 12: Nourishing Your Fasts

Macros Matter: What to Prioritize on Eating Days

Remember that what you eat during your eating windows has a big effect on your health as a whole. Your fasting times are very effective, but they work best when you don't eat too much on the days you don't fast.

What Do Macros Do?

"Macros" stands for "macronutrients," which are the three main nutrients your body needs in big amounts:

These are the building blocks of cells, muscles, enzymes, and other things. You can think of them as the building blocks of a healthy body.

• Carbs: These are your main power source. But not every carb is the same! Soon, we'll talk about the important changes.

• Fats: Healthy fats are important for making hormones, keeping cells working, brain health, and even energy, if you're fat-adapted.

Why macros are important when you're fasting

Picking the right macro mix for the days you eat is important for many reasons, including:

• Getting the most out of fasting: What you eat can either boost or weaken the good changes that fasting brings about in your cells.

• Helps Keep Muscles Strong: Eating enough protein while fasting is important for building and keeping muscle mass, which is good for your health and digestion.

• Managing Hunger and Energy: Eating a healthy diet of macros helps keep your blood sugar stable, which stops energy crashes and extreme hunger that can ruin your fasts.

• Improving your overall health: macros have an effect on your brain health, your energy levels, and even your happiness. Finding the right mix can help you feel your best over time.

Protein First: Your Best Friend for Fasting

When you eat, and especially when you fast, protein should be your main focus. This is why:

• Muscle Builder: Protein gives your body amino acids that it needs to build and heal muscle tissue. This is very important to keep you from losing muscle while you're fasting.

• Signal of Satiety: Protein makes you feel full and helps you control your hunger during fasting times.

• Metabolic Boost: Protein helps keep your metabolism healthy because it burns more calories than carbs or fats.

• Stabilizer for blood sugar: Protein slows down the intake of carbs, which stops blood sugar from going up and down too quickly, which drains your energy.

When you break your fast, try to eat some high-quality protein at every meal. Some examples are eggs, fish, chicken, beans, lentils, Greek yogurt, nuts, tofu, and so on.

Get Smart About Your Carbs

Carbohydrates give you energy, but what kind you eat is very important:

• Pay attention to complex carbs. Legumes, beans, whole grains, and vegetables give you long-lasting energy, fiber, and important nutrients. Don't eat refined carbs like white bread, sweets, and other foods that make your blood sugar rise.

• The Power of Fiber: Carbs that are high in fiber slow processing, make you feel full, and help keep your gut healthy, all of which are good for your brain and mood in a roundabout way!

• Watch Your Carbs: If you want to lose weight or are insulin resistant, watch how many carbs you eat. But there's no need to get rid of them totally, especially those healthy vegetables!

Do not be afraid of healthy fats.

They are necessary for your brain and body to work well while you're fasting.

• Boosts Satiety: Fats make you feel full, which eases hunger pangs that come from not eating for a while.

• Brain Fuel: Healthy fats are great for your brain. For a brain boost, eat nuts, seeds, avocados, olive oil, fatty fish, and olives.
• Source of energy: Healthy fats give you long-lasting energy during fasts if your body is "fat-adapted," which means it burns fat efficiently for fuel.

• Boosts flavor: Fats make healthy, whole foods taste great and fill you up, which is important for long-term health.

It's all about balance, says the motivation corner.

It takes some fine-tuning and self-awareness to find the right macro split for you. Here's how to make a custom plan that helps you feel your best and get the most out of fasting:

• Pay attention to your body. Notice how you feel after eating meals high in carbs vs. meals high in protein. Pay attention to how your energy changes when you eat different things.

• Track and Adjust: For a few weeks, keep an eye on your macros with a food record or journal. Change your balance based on how you feel, how long you can hold a pose, and what happens.

• Focus on Whole Foods: No matter what your ideal macro split is, eating whole, unprocessed foods is always the best way to be healthy and successful at fasting.

Examples of Meals That Will Help You Fast

Need some ideas? Here are some meal ideas that will help you reach your goals:

• For a high-protein breakfast, try scrambled eggs with spinach and feta, oatmeal with nuts and berries, or a green shake with protein.

• Lunch that is good for you: a big salad with grilled chicken, tuna, and whole-grain bread, or lentil soup with vegetables on the side.

• Dinner that fills you up: salmon with roasted vegetables, a bowl of rice and black beans, or a stir-fry of vegetables with tofu. **It's not a free pass to fast.**

Keeping your body hydrated and keeping your electrolytes in check

Food isn't the only thing that keeps us alive. Making sure you have enough water and electrolytes makes a HUGE difference in how you feel during your eating times and while you're fasting.

Let's talk about why these are so important for your health and your ability to fast.

Why staying hydrated is a must

About 60% of your body is water, which is important for many things! Why it's important to stay hydrated:

• Energy and Focus: Being even slightly dehydrated can make you feel brain fog, tired, and give you headaches, all of which are bad for a fast!

• Cleansing of cells: Water helps flush out toxins and waste, which supports the body's natural cleaning processes that happen when you fast.

• How to Deal with Hunger: What you think is hunger is actually thirst. Keep drinking water to avoid urges and hunger pangs.

• Healthy Metabolism: Staying properly hydrated is important for all of your body's systems to work well, including your metabolism.

The Link Between Electrolytes

Electrolytes are chemicals that your body needs and that have an electric charge. They are very important for:

• Fluid Balance: Electrolytes, such as sodium and potassium, help control how fluid moves around in your body, which affects how hydrated you are.

• How Muscles Work: Electrolytes are needed for muscle movements and your heartbeat. Not having the right balance can lead to cramps, weakness, and even heart rate problems.

• Nerve Signaling: Electrolytes help your nervous system send information. Some of the things your nervous system does are move your muscles and think clearly.

This is because when you fast, you normally lose more electrolytes through urine. To avoid tiredness, confusion, and other unpleasant symptoms, it is important to keep them up.

Key Electrolytes to Pay Attention To

To keep your balance while fasting, pay attention to:
• Sodium: Most people eat too much sodium on a daily basis, but it's easy to not get enough sodium when you fast. It's very important for nerve and muscle activity and the balance of fluids.

• Potassium: Keeps your muscles moving well and controls your heartbeat. Potassium levels can drop when you fast, which can make you feel weak and tired.

• Magnesium is needed for a huge number of body functions, such as making energy, keeping blood sugar levels steady, and reacting to stress. A lack of magnesium can make those headaches worse when you're fasting!

How to Stay Hydrated AND Get the Most Out of Your Electrolytes

Are you ready to make sure your body has everything it needs to grow and stay healthy? How to do it:

• Drink Smart: Water is the best thing you can do to help you fast! Aim for two to three liters every day. If you get bored with plain water, you can make it taste better by adding cucumber, mint leaves, or a squeeze of lemon.

• Help from herbs: Herbal teas that don't contain caffeine naturally keep you hydrated and give you an extra boost of plant chemicals that are good for your health.

• An electrolyte infusion of bone broth, coconut water, or electrolyte-enhanced water can help your body get back to normal during longer fasts.

• "Salty" Solutions: Adding a pinch of Himalayan pink salt or high-quality sea salt to your water can help you get the sodium you need during long fasts.

• Food Matters: On days when you eat, choose foods that are high in potassium, like bananas, avocados, spinach, and sweet potatoes.

Inspirational Corner: It's About Being Your Best!

People who fast often feel headaches, muscle cramps, and confusion, which are all signs that they are dehydrated or have an electrolyte imbalance. By putting electrolytes and staying hydrated first, you give yourself the power to stay refreshed, focused, and enjoy the process even more.

Pay attention to your body.

Your own wants may be different. Make the right choice by following these steps:

• Activity Is Important: If you work out hard or sweat a lot, you'll probably need more electrolytes to replace what you've lost.

• Don't Force It: Drinking too much water can also be bad for you. Follow your thirst; taking small sips often is better than drinking a lot all at once.

• Notice the Difference: Compare how you feel when you get enough water and minerals to how you feel when you don't. It will be easy to tell the difference!

Special Things to Think About

• Longer Fasts: If you go without food for more than 24 hours, you need to pay more attention to replacing your electrolytes to avoid bad effects.

• Medical Conditions: If you have problems with your kidneys, heart, or other parts of your body, you should always talk to your doctor about staying hydrated and getting enough fluids while fasting.

Water and electrolytes aren't just for your pleasure during fasts; they are also very good for your health in the long run. When you drink water or eat foods that are high in electrolytes, you give your body what it needs to work at its best, inside and out.

Stars of "Brain Food" to Include

Food is more than just calories. Some nutrients are like rocket fuel for your brain, protecting brain cells, improving mood, and improving your memory. By carefully including these foods, you not only get the most out of your eating days, but you also get the most out of your fasts.

Group 1: Omega-3 Powerhouses

It is important for your brain to have omega-3 fatty acids. Some studies show that these acids may help with memory, cognitive function, and even lowering the risk of cognitive loss that comes with getting older.

• Salmon, sardines, mackerel, walnuts, flaxseeds, and chia seeds are some of the best sources.

• Sneaky Ways to Boost: Sprinkle a few nuts and seeds on top of oatmeal, soups, or salads. Grind some flaxseed and add it to yogurt for extra omega-3s.

Group 2: Antioxidants with bright colors

Stress can damage cells in our brains. Antioxidants help protect cells!

Eat a lot of colorful fruits and veggies to get a strong dose of these antioxidants.

• Berry Power: Berries like blueberries, raspberries, and others are full of strong antioxidants. Eat them as a snack, mix them into your yogurt in the morning, or make smoothies with them.

• A Variety of Vegetables: For a wide range of vitamins that are good for your brain, eat broccoli, bell peppers, carrots, and leafy greens like spinach and kale.

• Spice It Up: Turmeric and ginger, among other herbs and spices, are also very good for you because they are strong antioxidants and reduce inflammation.

Group 3: Protein Power

We've already talked about how important protein is for fasting, but let's go into more detail about brain-friendly foods. Our brains need amino acids, which are found in protein, to make neurotransmitters, which are chemicals that affect our mood, focus, and ability to think.

• Choose lean foods like fish, chicken, beans, lentils, and tofu for good amino acid profiles and long-lasting energy.

• Omega-3 Combo: Fatty fish is great because it has both lean protein and those important omega-3s.

Group 4: Link Between Gut and Brain

There's a strong link between gut health and brain health. Here's how to take care of both:

• Fermented foods: Low-sugar yogurt with live active cultures, sauerkraut, or kimchi can help your gut bacteria stay healthy, which may have an effect on your brain function and happiness.

• Prebiotic Power: Foods like bananas, onions, garlic, and whole oats are prebiotic and feed the "good" bacteria in your gut.

Group 5: Good fats for you

Yes, good fats are important during your eating windows even when you're fasting!

• Avocados: These creamy treats are full of healthy fats and fiber, which help keep your blood sugar stable and give you long-lasting energy. This is important for staying focused.

• Nuts and seeds: easy to carry, filling, and full of brain-boosting nutrients like omega-3s and vitamin E.

• Olive oil: a tasty fat that helps reduce inflammation that you can add to salads or drizzle over cooked vegetables.

Motivation Corner: It's About Making Healthy, Tasty Choices

It doesn't have to be boring or hard to eat well for your brain. Try new recipes, look for seasonal foods, and get creative in the kitchen. The more fun these "brain food" superstars are, the more likely you are to make them a regular part of your life.

The Power of Fasting

Don't forget that these brain-friendly foods can boost the benefits of fasting:

• Cognitive Boost: Giving your brain the right nutrients may help you focus, think clearly, and feel the possible neuroprotective benefits of fasting.

• Helps with blood sugar: Eating a lot of whole foods that are high in fiber and lean protein can help keep your blood sugar in check, which will make both your fasting and eating windows easier to handle.

• Less inflammation: Eating foods that are high in antioxidants and low in inflammation may make the benefits of fasting even stronger, which is good for your brain's health and well-being as a whole.

Past the Plate

Not only the food you eat, but also the way you live can boost the benefits of your "brain food":

• Sleep: Not getting enough sleep will ruin all of your efforts to eat healthily. Make sure you get enough good quality rest to get the most out of your brain.

• Managing stress: Long-term stress is bad for the brain. Mindfulness and relaxation methods can help you eat well and stay healthy.

• Exercise: Get moving! Exercise is good for both the body and the brain because it keeps the blood flowing well and may slow down brain aging.

Think of your meals as a chance to give your brain the best care possible! When you choose healthy whole foods, you're not only improving your health, but you're also investing in a stronger, more resilient mind that will last for years to come.

Are you ready to turn your "what should I eat?" times into tasty choices that will help you stick to your fast? This part isn't about diets; instead, it's about easy, healthy recipes and sample meal plans that will make your eating times more enjoyable and good for your brain.

Example meal plans and quick, healthy recipes

Remember that there is no one way to find the best way for you to eat and fast at the same time. Try new things and make changes based on your needs and tastes!

Sample Meal Plan: 16:8 Time Restricted Eating

Breakfast (Around 10 AM): Oatmeal with Berries and Nut Butter: Whole oats, mixed berries, nut butter of choice, a few seeds, and a sprinkle of cinnamon.

Lunch (Around 2 PM): Power Salad with Grilled Chicken: Leafy greens base, grilled chicken, cherry tomatoes, cucumbers, sliced avocado, and a light vinaigrette dressing.

Dinner (Around 6 PM): Baked Salmon with Roasted Veggies: Salmon fillet with herbs, olive oil, topped with roasted sweet potatoes, broccoli, and cauliflower.

Snacks if needed: Handful of nuts, plain yogurt with fruit, or a hard-boiled egg.

Sample Meal Plan: 20:4 OMAD

Breaking the Fast (Sole Meal of the Day): Lentil soup, large salad with mixed greens, olives, cucumber, tomatoes, grilled chicken or tofu, dressing with olive oil and balsamic vinegar. Small bowl of mixed berries with plain yogurt for a light dessert.

Recipe Spotlight: Simple, Nourishing, and Fast!

Here are a few easy ideas that prioritize the "brain food" superstars:

Recipe #1: Antioxidant-Packed Smoothie

Ingredients: Spinach, frozen mixed berries, plain yogurt, a scoop of protein powder (optional), chia or flax seeds, water or unsweetened almond milk.

Instructions: Blend it all together, adjusting the liquid to your desired consistency. This is perfect for a quick and nutrient-dense breakfast or post-workout snack.

Recipe #2: Sheet Pan Salmon and Veggies

Ingredients: Salmon fillet, broccoli, bell peppers, olive oil, lemon juice, herbs and spices (like garlic, paprika, salt, and pepper).

Instructions: Veggies and salmon on a sheet pan, drizzle with olive oil, lemon, and spices. Bake at 400°F until cooked through. Easy, minimal cleanup, and bursting with flavor!

Recipe #3: Egg and Veggie Scramble

Ingredients: Eggs, onion, mushrooms, spinach, olive oil, turmeric, salt, and pepper.

Instructions: Crack and whisk eggs. Sauté onions, mushrooms, and spinach in a little olive oil. Add scrambled eggs and cook until firm. Sprinkle with turmeric for an extra anti-inflammatory boost.

Motivation Corner: It's About Sustainable Enjoyment

These are just starting points! Here's how to make this enjoyable and support those long-term healthy habits:

Flavor is King: Find simple recipes that use herbs and spices to add layers of deliciousness to those whole food staples.

Batch Prep: Cook a large batch of protein (chicken, lentils, tofu, etc.) and prep some veggies during the weekend to have healthy meal components ready to grab during the week.

Don't Be Afraid of Frozen and Canned: Frozen veggies are convenient and just as nutritious as fresh ones! Canned beans and lentils are a pantry staple for easy protein.

Embrace Simplicity: Some days, a simple piece of fruit and a handful of nuts is perfectly fine. Don't overcomplicate healthy eating!

Additional Resources to Inspire You

Here's where you can discover even more delicious ideas:

Websites: Look for sites that focus on whole foods, simple recipes, and brain-healthy eating.

https://www.lowcarbmaven.com/contact/, https://www.dietdoctor.com/ are some good places to start.

Cookbooks: Invest in a few cookbooks focused on healthy, whole-food cooking. Look for options that emphasize the nutrients we've talked about for brain health.

Online Communities: Join social media groups or forums where people share their healthy fasting, and meal prep tips, and recipes.

A Gentle Reminder

Your eating windows are NOT about undoing all the good work of your fasts. Instead, think of it as deeply nourishing both your body and brain to reap the maximum benefit from those strategic periods without food.

Chapter 13: Troubleshooting and Staying Motivated

Addressing Common Side Effects (Hunger, Headaches, etc.)

Even though fasting can be very helpful, it's normal to have some side effects as your body gets used to it.

What's good? These usually only last for a short time, and there are ways to lessen their effects or get rid of them completely!

Let's look at some of the most popular ones and give you the tools you need to handle them with ease.

Challenge #1: Dealing with Hunger Pangs

It's normal to feel hungry, especially in the beginning stages of fasting. Always keep in mind that your body is used to eating regularly! Here's how to deal with those signs of hunger:

• Stay hydrated: a lot of the time, what we think is hunger is just thirst. During your fasting time, drink water or herbal tea.

• Distractions that are planned: When you feel hungry, do something interesting, like going for a walk, calling a friend, or working on something interesting. Most of the time, they go away on their own.

• Change your thoughts: see your hunger as a good sign that your body is starting to burn fat. Think about how those fat stores are melting away with each pang!

• Mealtime Protein Power: During eating times, choose protein-rich foods first. It takes longer to feel full after eating protein.

• Gradual Progress: As your body gets used to the changes, hunger pangs usually get weaker. Begin with shorter fasts and build them up over time.

Challenge #2: Dealing with Headaches

Headaches that happen during fasting can be caused by changes in blood sugar levels, electrolyte issues, or not drinking enough water. Here's what you need to do:

• Salt Can Help: Adding a small amount of good sea salt or Himalayan salt to your water can help your body's fluids and ease headaches.

• Drink copious amounts of water—dehydration is a big cause! Pay attention to how much water you drink, especially at the beginning of your fasting time.

• Pay attention to your body. If headaches last a long time or are very bad, you should eat a healthy meal and try again the next day. It's important to rest and drink water.

• Helps Blood Sugar: If your headaches happen when your blood sugar drops, eating a handful of nuts during your mealtime can help keep your levels stable.

Challenge #3: Not having much energy

A lot of people feel more energetic when they fast, but you might feel a little tired some days. How to fix problems:

• Are you taking in enough food? Not eating enough during your eating windows can make you feel tired. Eat whole, healthy foods and don't be afraid of good fats!

• Check for Electrolytes: Electrolytes might help if you have headaches and low energy. It's amazing how helpful bone broth is here!

• What Time of Day It Is: Some people feel more energized when they work out during their fasting time. Try different things and see what works for you.

• You need to get enough sleep: Not getting enough sleep will make you less energetic, whether you are fasting or not. For best results, put peaceful sleep first.

Challenge #4: Having trouble sleeping

In a strange way, fasting can help many people sleep better, but at first, it can mess up their sleep habits.

• Timing is very important. Don't eat too close to sleep. Putting a few hours between your last meal and bedtime can help you sleep better.

• Calm Your Mind: Do something relaxing before bed to stop your mind from running, which could keep you from falling asleep.

• Magnesium Might Help: Magnesium can help you calm down. Before going to bed, try taking a vitamin or an Epsom salt bath.

Other Possible Side Effects and Ways To Fix Them

Some other brief side effects that happen less often are bad breath, changes in digestion, or irritability. Many times, bad breath goes away on its own, but you can help it along with sugar-free mint tea, brushing your teeth, and tongue cleaning.

If you're having stomach pain, make sure you break your fast with foods that are easy to digest. If you're feeling irritable, remember that it's just your body adjusting.

Take care of yourself by doing things like nature walks, light exercise, and your best ways to relax.

Corner for Motivation: It's Getting Easier!

It's important to remember that most of these side effects will go away as your body gets used to the new way of eating. When you fast successfully, your hungry pangs get weaker, your energy levels tend to stay the same, and your body turns into a fat-burning machine! Take your time and be kind to yourself.

Focus on the times when you feel calm, energized, and strong because you know you are in charge of your health and life.

Before starting a fasting plan, you should always talk to your doctor, especially if you have any specific worries or health problems. They can make specific suggestions to make sure you fast safely and successfully.

Remember that you may have to try different things to find the best fasting rhythm for YOUR body. Enjoy the process of getting to know yourself better, and use these possible side effects as helpful feedback to help you find a fasting practice that you can keep up, enjoy, and that works.

The benefits to your mind and body are worth the beginning changes!

Getting past slumps and setbacks

There will always be plateaus and failures on the way to a goal. It's the same for you as you fast! It's important to know that these short-term problems aren't failures, but rather chances to learn, adjust, and come out of them even stronger on your way to better health and longer life. Let's deal with those stops and starts one at a time.

The scale won't move on the plateau.

It happens a lot: you've been fasting regularly for a while and may have even lost some weight at first, but all of a sudden, the scale doesn't move. Here's what's going on and how to get past it:

• Muscle Is Important: If you work out, you may be building muscle while losing fat, which can make it look like you haven't made any progress on the scale.

• Don't just look at the number: Remember that fasting is good for more than just losing weight! Do your clothes fit you better now? How do you feel? Keep track of your progress or write down "how I feel" in your journal!

• It takes time to change body composition: It's not always easy to lose fat in a straight line, especially around trouble spots. Trust the process and enjoy the wins that aren't on a scale.

• Switch Things Up: Your body changes! You could try a slightly longer fasting period, a different eating time, or a different type of fasting all together.

Second Plateau Scenario: Mental and Emotional Stuckness

The plateaus can be more inside sometimes. Maybe the original rush of energy and clear thinking has worn off and left you in a more stable state. Or you haven't made any more progress since you lost those first few pounds. For these plateaus, you need to look for a different kind of problems:

• Digging Deeper: Bring your "why" back into focus. What made you decide to fast change? Do you need to make new goals to get yourself going again?

It's not a magic bullet to fast: Fasting is one tool, but it is very strong. Are there other areas (like sleep, stress control, etc.) that need more work to get the best results?

• Community Boost: Talk about your experience with a support group in person or on an internet forum. Hearing about other people's problems and successes can inspire you to do better.

• Refine, Don't Give Up: If your current fasting plan feels too rigid or unsatisfying, try different methods to find a rhythm that you can stick with.

Bad things: When Things Go Wrong in Life

Life will happen no matter how committed you are! Illness, travel, stressful events, or a full social schedule can all throw off your fasting plan for a while. To deal with losses with grace and strength, read on:

• Allow yourself to forgive: Feeling guilty or harsh on yourself is not helpful. Instead, accept that you made a mistake without being hard on yourself and think about how to get back on track.

• Keep an eye on the big picture: Your work won't be lost if you go off track for one day or even a week. Don't let it get so bad that you give up on all of your health goals.

• Make the switch slowly. If you've been fasting for a long time, start by doing shorter fasts more often to give your body time to get used to them again.

• Figure out what went wrong and learn from it. What caused you to break your routine? Knowing this helps you make plans for when things like this happen again.

The Corner for Motivation: Right now, this is just a process. Instead of a straight highway where every mile is the same, picture your fasting trip as a winding path with beautiful views.

Not all progress is straight lines, and it shouldn't be about being perfect all the time. That you choose to stick to those good habits over and over again is the most important thing.

Work on becoming more resilient. It's about finding out what works best for YOUR body, realizing that even short periods of fasting can be helpful, and understanding that each healthy choice you make makes your dedication to your health stronger.

Every week will be different, and some weeks will be easier than others. Sometimes you'll need to take a break before you can jump back in with renewed drive. All of that is part of the process! Remember that the seemingly ordinary times of choosing to feed your body and mind, like choosing to fast even when you're hungry or with other people, are what add up to a huge, long-lasting change.

Let reaching a peak make you want to try new things and improve your method. Accept setbacks as chances to be kind to yourself, which is a key skill for staying inspired over time.

The most important thing is to never forget how strong and flexible your mind and body are. They are your partners on this journey and can do more than you think they can with the right care.

How to Find Your Fasting Community and Build a Support System

Even though fasting has a lot of great possible benefits, it's important to remember that it can also cause some unique social problems. Having a support system can make all the difference in staying motivated and continuing this empowering practice for a long time, whether it's people who are trying to help you by giving you treats, family gatherings that revolve around food, or just feeling like you're not being understood

How to Handle Social Problems: It's Not Just Willpower

Being honest, even if you really want to say "no" to that sweet treat or to explaining your fasting plan for the hundredth time can be hard. In this case, using the power of the group is very helpful.

Do not forget that it is not only about effort. Studies have shown that having social support makes it much easier to stick to goals, deal with stress (which is good for fasting!), and just feel good about the choices we make.

Think about the people in your life who make you feel alive, important, and understood. This idea also refers to your practice of fasting. Being around people who "get it" or are actively working toward the same goals as you can help you stay strong when social pressure makes you doubt your resolve.

Where to Look to Find Your Fasting Crew

You don't have to do this by yourself, which is good news! Here's where you can find people who know what it's like to fast and celebrate your successes:

• Internet groups: Check out the many sites, such as Reddit, Facebook Groups, and even apps that are just for fasting, where people are sharing tips, helping each other with problems, and cheering each other on.

• Meet-ups in your area: Look around to see if there are any fasting groups nearby. They might set up social fasts, fitness things to do during fasts, or just a group to share potluck meals after a fast.

• Family, friends, and coworkers: You could be shocked! Talk about your fasting journey and offer help. Others may join you for shorter fasts, while others may become your biggest fans, even if they don't fully follow your lead.

• People who work in health care: If it makes sense, add your doctor or a chef who knows about fasting to your support team. It is very important to do this if you already have health problems or take medicines.

Things to Look For: How important it is to get the right kind of help

Not every kind of help is the same. Here's how to find a group that really makcs you fccl bcttcr:

• Positivity and support: Look for groups that focus on giving people power instead of criticism or competition. Celebrate all of your wins and accomplishments, no matter how big or small they are.

• Sharing knowledge: Find a group where people are willing to help you get past those temporary plateaus by giving you tips, troubleshooting ideas, and motivation.

• Fits Your Goals: If losing weight is your main goal, find a group whose main goal is the same as yours. If living a long time is important to you, look for people who feel the same way.

Getting Past Motivation: How Community Can Help You in Unexpected Ways

• Less loneliness: Knowing that other people "get it" makes you feel less alone, especially at social events that focus on food. When you tell a group of people who will support you about your goals, you're more likely to stick to those fasting times, even when things get tough.

• A broader view: Seeing other people's successes and failures gives you a good dose of reality and makes you more determined.

• Why being a mentor is fun: As you gain experience, helping newbies and paying it forward makes your own knowledge and dedication stronger.

Note: Finding the right balance between community and personal drive

Community is very helpful, but it's also important to find your own deep "why" for fasting and learn to rely on yourself. A long-term, healthy relationship with food is what it's all about, and you are always in charge of that trip! Don't become dependent on outside approval; instead, use your support system to boost your inner drive.

Corner for Motivation: Sharing a connection and a goal is important.

Finding a fasting group is mainly about remembering that making connections with other people helps you improve yourself. We all want to feel like we're being understood, and it's so empowering to talk about your problems and successes with people who are going through the same thing.

Imagine having someone you could talk to when you want to break your fast early but don't want to because they will remind you of why you started. Imagine how inspiring it would be to see someone complete a long fast that you've been trying to do, knowing that you can do it too.

People in your neighborhood are always there to remind you that you are not alone. They keep you motivated, give you useful advice, and add a little more joy to this empowering trip. In order to make your pledge to a healthier, more vibrant life stronger, go ahead and use your need to connect with others.

Chapter 14: Your Fasting Journey: Making it a Lifestyle

Listening to Your Body: Signs that Fasting is Working

It's not just about the end result when you fast; it's also about the trip that changes you along the way! You'll get a better sense of how fasting works for YOU if you learn to pay attention to your body's tiny and not-so-subtle signals.

These good changes can be very inspiring, keeping you committed to this way of life and showing you how it can improve your health and well-being in the long run.

The changes you see and feel in yourself and others are good signs that you're on the right path. When you are fasting, think of your body as a smart teacher. When you fast, you can adjust your method to get the most out of it by paying close attention to things like clearer thinking, balanced energy, or small changes in mood and appetite.

A sharper mind is one of the most exciting early signs that a lot of people notice. Your mind may feel clearer and less disorganized, which can help you concentrate on hard tasks or get through a busy workday without the normal brain fog distractions. A new sense of stable energy is another thing that many people feel.

Instead of the usual drops in blood sugar and cravings for a quick pick-me-up, you may find that your energy level stays higher all day. You may realize this when you realize you don't need as much coffee or sugary snacks to keep you going.

If we're talking about hunger, fasting might change the way you feel about food. As your body changes into a state where it burns fat efficiently, the strong wants for sugary or processed snacks usually start to go away. You might also become more aware of when you are really hungry. This makes it easier to tell the difference between real hunger and mindless eating, which is often caused by boredom or emotional triggers.

Your mood and health are affected by fasting in a bigger way.

Even though it's not a sure thing, a lot of people say that fasting makes them feel calmer, happier, and even less anxious. This could have something to do with the fact that your blood sugar levels are stable and inflammation is lower. Both of these things can have a big effect on how you feel every day.

Then there are changes in the outside world that add more good news. A big goal for many people is to lose weight or get rid of fat. If you want to get better at this, you may start to see changes in your body makeup, even if the scale won't move. Fasting can also help with health problems in a big way! It can help clear up your skin and give you a healthier glow by speeding up the autophagy process. Think of it as cellular spring cleaning.

You might even get benefits you didn't expect, like less bloating or better sleep, which is a huge step forward for both physical and mental recovery.

Notes and reminders: Not perfection, but progress

It's important to keep in mind that fasting has different effects on different people and that the time it takes to feel these benefits can vary.

Focus on praising your progress, even if it's just a small win. This will keep you going even more!

Small changes or days when you don't feel your best shouldn't get in the way of your spirit. Each person's journey is different, but the most important thing is to keep a positive attitude and see the good way you're going.

Keeping track of your events can be very helpful! The scale and measurements give you objective facts, but don't forget how useful a simple journal can be. Making notes about your energy, attention, mood, and any changes in your appetite can help you find patterns and reinforce those amazing changes inside that are easy to miss if you're only focused on losing weight.

It's not just about the number on the scale; fasting is about becoming healthy and more vital from the inside out. Fasting isn't just a short-term fix; it's a truly powerful lifestyle choice that will help you for years to come if you pay attention to your body and celebrate those real signs of progress.

Keeping track of progress beyond the scale: energy, mental clarity

It's time to stop being so focused on the scale!

Yes, losing weight or changing the way your body looks might have been the first reason you looked into fasting. But the truth is that this technique has benefits that go far beyond a number. You can make your health journey much more sustainable and satisfying by focusing on those big changes that will happen in your mental clarity, energy levels, mood, and general well-being.

You can think of it as adding new ways to track your progress. The scale gives you a specific piece of information, but keeping track of those less obvious (but just as important!) changes is like drawing a full picture of how fasting has changed your life. This increased knowledge gives you a strong motivational boost and encourages you to stick with this lifestyle for a long time.

So, where do you turn your attention? Start by clearing your mind. Is it easy for you to stay on task at work and not get distracted? Are you able to solve problems more quickly and with more focus? As you do more fasting, you'll notice that those times when you can't think straight happen less often.

Next, pay attention to how much energy you have. You make it through the day with less tiredness, so you don't need that extra cup of coffee in the afternoon. Knowing about these changes in energy makes it clearer why fasting can help you feel better every day.

You shouldn't forget about how it affects your mood either! A lot of people say that fasting makes them feel calmer, better able to handle stress, and maybe even less anxious. Stabilized blood sugar and less inflammation are two things that might have an effect on these changes. Both of these have a big effect on how you feel, both physically and mentally.

You should also look at how well you sleep and how you feel about food. Are you able to fall asleep faster and feel truly rested when you wake up? For both physical and mental health, this longer, restorative sleep is very important.

Also, pay attention to whether your strong desires for sweets, salty snacks, or random snacking start to fade. Fasting helps you have a better relationship with food by letting you tell the difference between real hunger and emotional or habitual eating triggers.

It's important to keep in mind that fasting doesn't always have clear effects at set times. Waves of progress are possible. Some people may feel a sudden surge of mental clarity and boundless energy right away, while others may see changes in their inflammatory conditions or body composition over a longer period of time.

This is why it's so important to have a way to keep track of these meaningful changes. A simple book can help you a lot! Take a few minutes every day to write down any good changes you notice in your focus, energy, mood, sleep, and anything else.

You could also "Rate Your Day" by giving yourself a number from 1 to 10 based on things like your overall energy or how well your emotions are balanced. After a while, you'll start to see patterns.

For example, did you feel extra alert after a 20-hour fast? Did a certain type of meal on the day you ate seem to affect how well you focused the next day? With these specific insights, you can make small changes to your fasting routine to get the most out of it. It's most exciting to keep track of your progress in this all-around way because it makes you value fasting even when the numbers on the scale don't move as quickly as you'd like. When you feel more mentally clear, your energy is balanced, or your mental health is better, it's a powerful reminder of why you chose this path in the first place.

Accepting those wins that don't have to do with the scale will keep you motivated, which will lead to lasting change and a stronger connection with your body's amazing ability to heal and grow.

Long-term changes in how you think and how to make fasting last

The most powerful thing about fasting is that it can change how you feel about food, your health, and your body. That's not even close to what it's about. By making certain changes to the way you think, you can use fasting as a long-term tool to help you reach your goals and improve your health for years to come.

Shift #1: From Limitations to Freedom

Getting over the idea that fasting means not eating or drinking is one of the hardest things to do. But if you do things the right way, it's actually the opposite! Instead of thinking about what you can't have, pay attention to how good you feel when you're fasting. Enjoy your clearer mind, steady energy, and feeling of being light in your body. This change from being limited to being free is important for making fasting feel like fun instead of something you have to suffer.

Shift #2: Hunger Is Not an Enemy

People often teach us to be afraid of being hungry, so as soon as we start to feel hungry, we reach for a snack. When you fast, you learn to see hunger as a good sign from your body.

Paying attention to these signs of hunger helps you get a better sense of what your body really needs. It might surprise you to learn that those hunger pangs often go away, showing that they were caused by habit or boredom instead of a real need for food.

Shift #3: Food as Fuel, Not entertainment

When you fast, you stop mindlessly snacking and using food as a treat or to take your mind off of things. Instead, you start to see those times to eat as chances to really feed your body. When you're really hungry, you're more deliberate about what you eat and want whole, nutrient-dense foods instead of processed treats that you want on a whim. This is a change toward enjoying the food you eat and getting the most nutrition out of it.

Shift #4: Flexibility Is Better Than Rigidity

Being flexible is important for long-term success because life happens. Don't let a social event or a sudden change in your plans stop you from moving forward. If you want to avoid feeling guilty or giving up, just change your fasting time or your plan for that day. Enjoy being able to adapt to the unpredictable nature of life without giving up on your general commitment to health and well-being.

Shift #5: Being patient and kind to yourself

It takes time to change! Don't expect miracles to happen overnight; instead, enjoy the trip and focus on the steady progress. When it feels harder to fast some days, be kind to yourself. Instead of being hard on yourself, be kind to yourself and remember that every time you decide to start a fast, you're getting stronger.

Every little win is worth celebrating, whether it's an extra hour added to your fast, clearer thinking, or the power to say no to those old eating urges.

Getting it to stick: Tips for Being Sustainable

• Start small and get used to it: Don't feel like you have to start long fasts right away. Start by fasting for shorter periods of time more often. As you get used to it, slowly increase the length and number of times you fast. Being consistent is more important than doing great things every once in a while.

• Get into the groove: Try different ways of fasting to find the one that works best for you. Is it eating at set times every day? A few times a week, longer fasts? No one-size-fits-all method works! How does your body react to different things? Find out what works for you.

• Pay attention to "Why": When you start to lose motivation, remember why you started this trip in the first place. Was it to improve your health markers, get that feeling of having endless energy back, or deal with a long-term health problem? Picture yourself reaching those goals, and let that drive you to do your best.

• Helping the community: Find a community that will help you, whether it's an online group or a friend who feels the same way. Sharing your experiences, problems, and small wins can help you stay motivated and make you feel less alone.

Remember that progress doesn't always happen in a straight line. There will be days when old habits come back, failures, and plateaus. That is totally normal!

Realizing that these are just temporary problems and always going back to the core attitude changes that make fasting a healthy habit that lasts and gives you power are what gives it its real power.

And each fasting time that goes by makes you more confident in your body's natural ability to heal and grow. Think about how that will feel in a month or a year. That's the real magic of living this way of life!

Chapter 15: The Brain-Healthy Future You

Recap of Key Benefits of Fasting for the 40+ Brain

When we get to our 40s, 50s, and beyond, it's more important than ever to take care of our brains. What's good? Fasting has become a strong way to protect your brain health as you age and may even help your brain work better and lower your risk of age-related decline. Let's go over the amazing benefits you've learned about and talk about why they're so great for keeping your brain strong and sharp throughout your life.

Cellular cleaning on high gear

Think back to autophagy. It's how your cells get rid of broken proteins, parts that don't work right, and other "junk" that's inside the cell. As you get older, this process naturally slows down. Fasting gives your brain cells a big boost, like a deep clean.

Getting rid of this built-up junk makes your brain work better and makes it less likely that the misfolded proteins linked to Alzheimer's and Parkinson's will build up.

Neurogenesis: Making New Neurons for a Young Brain

The fact that fasting can raise levels of BDNF, a brain growth factor that helps new brain cells form, is one of the most exciting finds! This increased neurogenesis could lead to better learning, memory, and defense against the "shrinkage" of the brain that comes with getting older.

Inflammation Buster

A lot of diseases that come with getting older, like brain fog and cognitive loss, are caused by chronic inflammation. When you fast, your body naturally fights inflammation, which stops this harmful process in your brain and body. When your brain is calm and less swollen, you can think more clearly, feel better, and be healthier all around.

Focus and mental agility

A lot of people say that fasting makes their minds clearer and helps them concentrate. This might be partly because the body is turning to making ketone bodies for energy and also because fasting generally makes the brain feel calmer. This improved mental edge is a game-changer whether you're juggling a demanding job, dealing with changed family dynamics, or finding new hobbies after retirement.

Possible Protection Against Neurodegeneration

Even though more studies with real people are needed to be sure, there is strong evidence that fasting may help lower the chance of or slow the progression of diseases like Alzheimer's, Parkinson's, and Huntington's.

We can feel hopeful and strong as we get closer to the ages when neurological diseases become more common.

After the Metabolic Reset

Fasting has effects on more than just the brain. Its powerful effects on improving insulin sensitivity, improving metabolic health, and encouraging fat loss protect our brain cells in a roundabout way. Consider it as optimizing your whole body, which creates a better space for your brain to grow.

Things you should think about before you start

Even though the possible benefits are very exciting, here are some things to keep in mind:

• See your doctor: Before starting a new fasting plan, it's very important to talk to your doctor, especially if you are over 40, already have a health problem, or take medicine. They can help you make a plan that is safe and works.

• Start slowly and pay close attention: Start by fasting for shorter periods of time more often, and then build up based on how you feel. Pay attention to what your body is telling you and make changes as needed.

•It's a Way of Life, Not a Quick Fix: The real power of fasting is in how often you do it. Make it a long-term part of your health routine to get long-lasting brain-boosting effects.

A Word About Hope and Strength

Findings about fasting and brain health that make us feel in charge are some of the most energizing things about them. Even though biology and getting older play a part, the choices you make about your lifestyle have a huge effect on your brain's health and development. When you fast, YOU are in charge of your brain health.

As you get older, imagine being sure that you've done everything you could to keep that amazing command center in your head safe. Think about what you could do if you had a better memory, lasting mental speed, and a mind that was ready to take on everything life has to offer.

When you fast and practice other healthy habits, you're investing in the best form of yourself in the future. And the journey starts right now.

How to Keep Your Brain Healthy for Good

You now know how fasting can help your brain health in amazing ways, but let's not forget the power of other tools that work together to make those benefits even stronger! You can think of this as creating your own unique brain-health defense system.

This is a multifaceted method that gives you the power to safeguard, nourish, and improve your brain health for years to come.

Tool #1: Giving your brain food

Even though fasting gives your body a break from digestion, you should still think about what you eat when you do allow yourself to eat. Here are the main parts of a food that will help your brain:

• Pay attention to whole foods: Choose whole grains, legumes, nuts, seeds, and colored fruits and vegetables first. These give you important nutrients, vitamins, and fiber that help your brain work well.

• Fats that are good for you are important: Fish with a lot of fat, avocados, olive oil, and nuts all have omega-3s and other brain-healthy fats that keep neurons healthy and reduce swelling.

• Lean Protein Power: Choose lean protein sources like fish, chicken, beans, and other animals to give your brain the building blocks it needs to make neurotransmitters and keep cells healthy overall.

• Reduce the number of offenders: Cut back on prepared foods, too much sugar, and fats that are bad for you. These make inflammation and reactive stress worse, which goes against your efforts to keep your brain healthy.

Tool #2: The Power of Moving Around

Regular exercise isn't just good for your body; it's also great for your brain! It's important to work out because:

• More blood flow: exercise sends oxygenated, nutrient-rich blood to your brain, which helps it work better now and in the future.

• BDNF Boost: Do you remember that brain food? One of the best natural ways to stimulate it is to be active!

• Neurogenesis and Memory: Some research shows that exercise may help neurons grow, especially in the hippocampus, which is an important part of the brain for learning and remembering.

• Stress-Relieving: Working out lowers stress hormones, which makes your brain work better in a calmer setting.

• Try different things: Do things you really enjoy! Any kind of exercise will work as long as you do it regularly, whether it's brisk walks, dancing, swimming, or yoga.

Tool #3: Learning How to Handle Stress

Long-term worry is very bad for brain health. To protect your brain health and general well-being, you need to find healthy ways to deal with stress.

• Mindfulness Is Important: Even short sessions of mindful meditation can help lower stress, improve focus, and build mental strength.

• Spending time in nature: Being in green areas, sunlight, and fresh air can naturally calm you down and lower your stress hormones.

To quickly get your nervous system out of "fight or flight" mode and into a relaxation reaction, try deep breathing exercises.

• Make restorative sleep a priority. Getting enough sleep is essential for brain health; it's when memory consolidation and cell repair happen.

Tool #4: Making your mind work harder

Working out your mind is just as important for brain health as working out your body. It's kind of like strength training for your brain networks. To keep your brain sharp, do these things:

• Lifelong Learning: Taking on new tasks, like learning a new language, an instrument, or a subject that interests you, keeps your brain flexible and ready to use.

• Puzzles and brain games: Do things that use a variety of cognitive skills. For example, Sudoku, crosswords, and even strategy video games can help your brain stay in shape.

• Social Connection: Having strong social ties may lower the chance of cognitive decline. Have deep talks and look for groups where you can feel connected and inspired.

Tool #5: fasting as your main pillar

The research is interesting, and your own experience may already show that going without food for long amounts of time is good for your brain. Now it's time to find YOUR fasting rhythm so that it becomes a constant part of your life:

• Try something: If this feels good for your body, start with shorter fasts that happen more often and work your way up to longer ones that happen less often.

• Pay attention to your body: Change your fasting plan based on how you feel, how much energy you have, and when you start to feel hungry. You need to be flexible!

• Nourishing Windows: It's best to combine fasting with a brain-healthy meal to get the most out of it and avoid bingeing during those times.

The Corner for Motivation: This trip is very exciting!

Putting together a brain health toolkit isn't about following strict rules; it's about making useful findings! Fun and long-lasting are very important. Try different things until you find what makes your body and mind feel great, and be proud of your dedication to taking care of that amazing organ that guides you through life.

Remember that over time, even small steps in the right way can build up to big ones. Think about yourself in 5, 10, or even 20 years, when you have a sharp mind, a strong memory, and the mental energy to handle life's events. This is the promise of putting brain health first, and the path starts today with the choices you make!

Of course! Here is a draft of the "Inspiring Call to Action" part, which is meant to give the reader power and drive. Please let me know if you'd like a certain point to be emphasized more!

Inspiring Call to Action: Trust the Strength of Being in Charge

During this trip, you've learned a lot about your brain, including its amazing abilities, its weaknesses, and most importantly, the amazing things you can do to change its health. This is about more than just information; it's about change. You can become more aware of the fact that you have more power over your brain health and general health than you ever thought possible.

Brain health and getting older have been talked about as if they were inevitable for far too long. People tell us that memory loss, mental fog, and less mental power are all normal parts of getting older. But new and exciting studies on fasting, nutrition, lifestyle, and the potential of neuroplasticity is breaking down that old story! Genetics and age do play a part, but science shows that the choices we make have a much bigger effect on how our brains work and change over time.

This change in point of view is nothing less than freeing. You don't have to feel like a helpless passenger as the years go by. You can take charge of your brain health and feel positive about it. Picture yourself ten years from now. What kind of sharpness, energy, and clarity of mind do you want to have?

What does it feel like to have a good memory, be able to learn new things without much trouble, and be able to enjoy every part of life with a mind that lets you do well? Remember that the power to make your vision come true starts today, with every choice you make, every time you fast, and every step you take toward a brain-healthy living.

Remember that there is no one "right" way to do things. Your brain health kit will be just for you! Someone else might do better with shorter fasts every day, while you might do better with longer fasts a few times a week.

A long walk in the woods might help you relax, and your best friend might find that dancing puts her in a happy flow state that is good for her brain. The beauty is in the process of finding things on your own.

This trip is both an in-depth look at yourself and an exciting adventure. Watch how different things make you feel and how they help you concentrate. Watch how your mental energy changes when you change the length of your fasts. Check to see if some types of exercise help you in more ways than one. Which things make you happy, lower your stress, and make you feel full of life? Focus on those things and make them a big part of your plan to take care of not only your body but also your brain, which is the most complicated and amazing organ you have.

There will no doubt be days when things are easier than others. This is where having a strong "why" and a neighborhood come in handy. Find people who share your interests and can help and inspire you.

When you lose motivation, think back to the main reason you started this journey in the first place. It could have been a desire to live a long, healthy life with the people you love or a desire to stop brain decline that you saw in family members.

Use your "why" to drive you to succeed.

Think about what you could do if you had a healthy, strong brain that would help you through the years to come. Making your brain health a priority can help you finally go after your dreams, make stronger connections, and finish creative projects.

Remember that every time you choose to fast strategically, eat whole foods to fuel your body, laugh with friends and family, or give yourself a mental challenge with a new Sudoku game, you are building a future full of mental agility and long-lasting cognitive vitality.

This journey may start with learning about the science, but what really changes things is putting what you've learned into practice! What are you going to do next? Are you going to attempt a 16-hour fast for the first time? Instead of looking through your phone after dinner, why not go for a quick walk outside? Look into a new meal that's full of those "brain food" stars. Every step moves you forward, no matter how small it is.

Since the day you were born, your brain has been there for you. At this point, it's your job to care for and help it.

This is your inspiring call to action: take charge of your mental health, believe in the empowering science, and make the future one where your mind is your most reliable partner on all the adventures that lie ahead.

Conclusion
Your Extraordinary Journey Begins

So, dear reader, this exploration is over. But your real journey—the one that will change you the most—is just starting! You are no longer just a bystander when it comes to your health, your life, and most importantly, the health of your brain, which is the amazing control center inside your head.

You now have strong tools and information at your disposal. You've gone into the world of cells and learned about the complicated processes that fasting starts to heal and rejuvenate you.

You now understand the strong connection between the foods you eat and not only your physical health but also your mental health, happiness, and ability to think and remember things. You now know that exercise, dealing with stress, and those times when you learn through play have a big impact on how your brain works and how long it lasts.

The most important thing is that you were aware of how much power you have to change your life, from your mental flexibility to your metabolic health.

This book is like an insightful tour guide that showed you the most beautiful and rejuvenating places to visit. Now it's time to put on your shoes and go on an adventure! This is about taking action, trying new things, and figuring out what makes YOU feel alive, motivated, and mentally strong.

You could start your fasting trip with a few simple time-limited eating windows per week. As your body and mind get used to it, you can slowly increase the length and frequency of your fasts.

You might become an adventurous cook and find the joy and flavor explosion in brain-boosting, whole-food meals that make you feel full and nourished.

Putting on your sneakers and exploring nature walks is one option. Another is to put on some music and dance. This may awaken something in your body and soul that is also good for your brain.

Remember that living a long, healthy, and mentally satisfying life isn't just about getting older. It's about how you feel along the way and having the mental and physical strength to take advantage of all the options and deal with the problems that will inevitably arise.

Knowing that the decisions you make every day can affect your health and mental well-being for years or even decades to come gives you a lot of power. Imagine being full of energy five or ten years from now, able to handle difficult work projects with ease, or finally learning that language you've always wanted to speak.

Think about how confident you'll be as you get older if you know you did everything you could to build a body and mind that will help you, not hold you back. That's the possibility you've unlocked by reading these pages and getting ideas from them.

It won't always be easy on this road, and it shouldn't be about being ideal. Life is unexpected, and there will be days when old temptations come back or when you can't sleep. But don't let those short-term slip-ups get you down! You're truly empowered when you can change your path, re-center, and go back to the things that you know make a difference in your health.

Get help from groups of people who share your interests, both online and off.

Celebrate your wins, whether they're the extra energy you have after a 20-hour fast, how easy it is to learn a new skill, or just how your mind feels calmer and stronger when life gets stressful. Also, remember to be patient and nice to yourself. It takes time for real change to happen.

With the passing of time, you'll continue to learn, change, and find new ways to make your fasting, food choices, and way of life better fit your changing needs. Allow your interest to guide you as new study comes out. This book can be seen as the start of a conversation with your body about how to heal, rejuvenate, and grow.

Believing in your body's amazing potential and the power of your choices to shape your bright future is the best gift you can give yourself. Accept the tools of fasting, eating foods that are good for your brain, moving around for fun, dealing with stress, and learning new things all the time...and let them help you become the strongest, healthiest, and most mentally tough person you can be at all times.

Right now, is the start of your amazing trip!